Keto Bread and Keto Snacks 2021

Easy-to-follow Ketogenic Diet Cookbook With Low-Carb and Gluten-Free Wheat Recipes For Beginners.

TABLE OF CONTENTS

INTRODUCTION

The keto diet is the high-fat, moderate-protein, super-low-carb craze you've probably read about online or heard your coworker rave about. And while it has helped countless people lose weight, the rules of what you can and can't eat are pretty restrictive.

In general, you should aim to eat fewer than 50 carbs a day to keep your body in the fat-burning state of ketosis. The general macro breakdown is 70 to 80 percent fat, 15 to 20 percent protein, and five to 10 percent carbs. Since carbs are present in many healthy, keto-friendly foods such as leafy, nonstarchy vegetables and low-sugar fruit, it's generally recommended to stay away from other grains and carb-heavy starches. Yes, this includes bread and all the beloved bread products. Luckily, there's a caveat.

"While traditional bread - yes, even whole wheat and whole grain - is too high in carbohydrates to include on a ketogenic diet, there are several great low-carb bread recipes and products that can be included if you miss the occasional sandwich or roll with your meal

WHAT IS KETOSIS?

The "keto" diet is any extremely low- or no-carbohydrate diet that forces the body into a state of ketosis.

Ketosis occurs when people eat a low- or no-carb diet and molecules called ketones build up in their bloodstream.

Low carbohydrate levels cause blood sugar levels to drop and the body begins breaking down fat to use as energy.

Ketosis is actually a mild form of ketoacidosis. Ketoacidosis mostly affects people with type 1 diabetes. In fact, it is the leading cause of death of people with diabetes who are under 24 years of age.

However, many experts say ketosis itself is not necessarily harmful.

Some studies, in fact, suggest that a ketogenic diet is safe for significantly overweight or obese people.

However, other clinical reviews point out that patients on low-carbohydrate diets regain some of their lost weight within a year.

ARE KETO "CHEAT" FOODS HEALTHY?

One of the biggest hurdles of any diet, and especially the keto diet, is a deprivation mentality. If you believe you can't have something, you may find yourself craving it even more.

Keto "cheat" foods, proponents argue, may help you satisfy those longings while not blowing your carb budget.

Keto-friendly versions of foods can most certainly be a part of a balanced diet," said Amanda Maucere, a registered dietitian and nutritionist (RDN) for the Lung Health Institute.

These foods can also help people benefit from nutritional ketosis for a longer period of time without feeling deprived of the foods they are used to eating,

KETO BREAD RECIPES

1 LOW CARB GLUTEN FREE CRANBERRY BREAD

A delicious gluten free low carb cranberry bread with fresh cranberries. This sugar-free bread uses a combination of stevia and erythritol sweeteners.

Prep Time 10 minutes
Cook Time 1 hour 15 minutes
Total Time 1 hour 25 minutes
Servings 12 people

Ingredients

- 2 cups almond flour
- 1/2 cup powdered erythritol or Swerve, see
- Note 1/2 teaspoon Steviva stevia powder
- see Note 1 1/2 teaspoons baking powder
- 1/2 teaspoon baking soda
- 1 teaspoon salt

- 4 tablespoons unsalted butter melted (or coconut oil)
- 1 teaspoon blackstrap molasses optional (for brown sugar flavor)
- 4 large eggs at room temperature
- 1/2 cup coconut milk
- 1 bag cranberries 12 ounces

Instructions

- Preheat oven to 350 degrees; grease a 9-by-5 inch loaf pan and set aside.
- In a large bowl, whisk together flour, erythritol, stevia, baking powder, baking soda, and salt; set aside.
- In a medium bowl, combine butter, molasses, eggs, and coconut milk.
- Mix dry mixture into wet mixture until well combined.
- Fold in cranberries. Pour batter into prepared pan.
- Bake until a toothpick inserted in the center of the loaf comes clean, about 1 hour and 15 minutes.
- Transfer pan to a wire rack; let bread cool 15 minutes before removing from pan.

Nutrition Info

Calories 179 Calories from Fat 135
Total Fat 15g 23%
Saturated Fat 4g 20%
Protein 6.4g 13%

---

2 MONKEY BREAD

Prep/Cook Time: 1 hour, 30 mins

Ingredients

DOUGH:

- 3 cup blanched almond flour (10 oz) (or 1 cup coconut flour or

5 oz)
- 10 TBS psyllium husk powder (no substitutes) (90 grams)
- 4 tsp baking powder
- 2 tsp Celtic sea salt
- 1 cup Swerve (or erythritol and 1 tsp stevia glycerite)
- 8 egg whites (16 whites if using coconut flour)
- 5 TBS apple cider vinegar (2 oz)
- 2 cup BOILING water (14 oz)

FILLING:

- 8 oz cream cheese

TOPPING:

- 8 TBS butter (or coconut oil)
- 1 TBS cinnamon
- 1/2 cup Swerve (or erythritol)

Instructions

- Preheat the oven to 375 degrees F. In a large bowl, combine the flour, psyllium powder (no substitutes: flaxseed meal won't work), baking powder, salt and sweetener. Mix until combined. Add in the eggs and vinegar and combine until a thick dough. Add boiling water into the bowl. Mix until well combined. When you add the water the dough will be very sticky but after mixing for a couple minutes it will firm up.

- Separate dough into 20 equal sized disks. You can spray some more spray on top of the dough to help keep it from sticking to your fingers. Cut cream cheese into 20 squares. Place on square on top of each dough disk and form the disk around the sides of the cream cheese.

- Place 10 of the squares in the bottom of a greased bundt pan with the cream cheese facing up. Sprinkle cinnamon and Swerve on top. Then put the remaining 10 squares inverted on top of the first 10 (making the cream cheese touch). Bake for

55 minutes.

Meanwhile, make the topping.

- Place all ingredients into a medium sized bowl and combine until smooth. After it has baked for 55 minutes, remove and quickly spread topping over the monkey bread. Return to oven and bake for 15 minute. Allow to cool for 20-30 minutes before turning over and removing from bundt pan. Makes 14 servings.

Nutrition Info

308 calories, 21.1g fat, 2.9g protein, 28.9 carbs, trace fiber (28.9g effective carbs)

---

3 LOW CARB HOT CROSS BUNS

Low-carb hot cross buns are perfect any time of the year. To ensure they bake evenly, ensure they are not too big and not too thick.

Prep Time15 mins
Cook Time20 mins
Total Time35 mins
Servings:4

Ingredients

- 60 g coconut flour
- 30 g psyllium husks
- 1 tsp baking powder
- 2 tbsp granulated sweetener of choice or more, to your taste

- 1/2 tsp salt
- 1/2 tsp mixed spice
- 1/2 tsp cinnamon
- 1/2 tsp ground cloves
- 4 eggs - medium
- 250 ml boiling water
- raisins/chocolate chips/ cacao nibs optional

Icing

- powdered sweetener icing mix

Instructions

Low Carb Hot Cross Buns

- Mix all the dry ingredients in a mixing bowl.
- Add the eggs and mix.
- Add the boiling water and mix until evenly combined.
- Roll into 8 equal balls and place on a baking tray.
- Bake in a fan assisted oven at 180C/350F for 20-30 minutes until golden on the outside and cooked in the centre.

Icing

- Mark each hot cross bun with a cross using the powdered sweetener confectioners/icing mix and water paste.

Nutrition Info

Calories 84 Calories from Fat 28
Total Fat 3.1g 5%
Total Carbohydrates 8.9g 3%
Dietary Fiber 6.8g 27%
Sugars 0.7g
Protein 5.6g 11%

---

4 KETO PUMPKIN BREAD

A delicious, moist, keto pumpkin bread full of warm spices and amazing pumpkin flavor. Made with almond and coconut flours to keep it healthy, gluten-free, and low-carb.

Prep Time: 10 minutes
Cook Time: 45 minutes
Total Time: 55 minutes
Serving: 10

Ingredients

- 1/2 cup butter, softened
- 2/3 cup erythritol sweetener, like
- Swerve 4 eggs large
- 3/4 cup pumpkin puree, canned (see notes for fresh)
- 1 tsp vanilla extract
- 1 1/2 cup almond flour
- 1/2 cup coconut flour
- 4 tsp baking powder
- 1 tsp cinnamon
- 1/2 tsp nutmeg
- 1/4 tsp ginger
- 1/8 tsp cloves
- 1/2 tsp salt

Instructions

- Preheat the oven to 350°F. Grease a 9"x5" loaf pan, and line with parchment paper.
- In a large mixing bowl, cream the butter and sweetener together until light and fluffy.
- Add the eggs, one at a time, and mix well to combine.
- Add the pumpkin puree and vanilla, and mix well to combine.
- In a separate bowl, stir together the almond flour, coconut flour, baking powder, cinnamon, nutmeg, ginger, cloves, salt. Break up any lumps of almond flour or coconut flour.
- Add the dry ingredients to the wet ingredients, and stir to combine. (Optionally, add up to 1/2 cup of mix-ins, like chopped nuts or chocolate chips.)
- Pour the batter into the prepared loaf pan. Bake for 45 - 55

minutes, or until a toothpick inserted into the center of the loaf comes out clean.

- If the bread is browning too quickly, you can cover the pan with a piece of aluminum foil.

Nutrition Info

Calories: 165 Total Fat: 14g Saturated Fat: 7g Unsaturated Fat: 4g Cholesterol: 99mg Sodium: 76mg Carbohydrates: 6g Fiber: 3g Sugar: 1g Protein: 5g

---

5 EASY PALEO KETO BREAD RECIPE - 5 INGREDIENTS

If you want to know how to make the BEST keto bread recipe, this is it! It makes fluffy white paleo bread that's quick & easy. Just 5 basic ingredients! Course Breakfast, Main Course, Side Dish

Prep Time 10 minutes
Cook Time 1 hour 10 minutes
Total Time 1 hour 20 minutes

Ingredients

Basic Ingredients

- 1 cup Blanched almond flour
- 1/4 cup Coconut flour
- 2 tsp Gluten-free baking powder
- 1/4 tsp Sea salt
- 1/3 cup Butter (or 5 tbsp + 1 tsp; measured solid, then melted; can use coconut oil for dairy-free)
- 12 large Egg white (~1 1/2 cups, at room temperature)

Optional Ingredients (recommended)

- 1 1/2 tbsp Erythritol (can use any sweetener or omit)
- 1/4 tsp Xanthan gum (for texture - omit for paleo)
- 1/4 tsp Cream of tartar (to more easily whip egg whites)

Instructions

- Preheat the oven to 325 degrees F (163 degrees C). Line an 8 1/2 x 4 1/2 in (22x11 cm) loaf pan with parchment paper, with extra hanging over the sides for easy removal later.
- Combine the almond flour, coconut flour, baking powder, erythritol, xanthan gum, and sea salt in a large food processor. Pulse until combined.
- Add the melted butter. Pulse, scraping down the sides as needed, until crumbly.
- In a very large bowl, use a hand mixer to beat the egg whites and cream of tartar (if using), until stiff peaks form. Make sure the bowl is large enough because the whites will expand a lot.
- Add 1/2 of the stiff egg whites to the food processor. Pulse a few times until just combined. Do not over-mix!

- Carefully transfer the mixture from the food processor into the bowl with the egg whites, and gently fold until no streaks remain. Do not stir. Fold gently to keep the mixture as fluffy as possible.

- Transfer the batter to the lined loaf pan and smooth the top. Push the batter toward the center a bit to round the top.

- Bake for about 40 minutes, until the top is golden brown. Tent the top with aluminum foil and bake for another 30-45 minutes, until the top is firm and does not make a squishy sound when pressed. Internal temperature should be 200 degrees. Cool completely before removing from the pan and slicing.

Nutrition Info

Calories 82
Fat 7g
Protein 4g
Total Carbs 3g
Net Carbs 1g
Fiber 2g

Sugar 1g

---

6 KETO BLUEBERRY LEMON BREAD

This recipe for keto blueberry bread is grain-free, gluten-free, sugar-free, low carb and it's diabetic and keto-friendly. If that's not enough it also happens to be easy to make.

Prep Time: 10 minutes
Cook Time: 1 hour
Additional Time: 15 minutes
Total Time: 1 hour 25 minutes
Serving: 12

Ingredients

Keto Blueberry Lemon Bread Batter

- 2 1/2 cups of finely milled almond flour
- 1 cup of sugar substitute
- 2 teaspoons of baking powder
- 1/2 teaspoon of sea salt
- 8 whole eggs
- 8 ounces of room temperature full-fat cream cheese
- 2 teaspoons of lemon extract
- 1/2 cup of room temperature unsalted
- butter 2 cups of fresh or frozen whole
- blueberries 1 tablespoon of lemon zest

Keto Lemon Glaze

- 3/4 cup of confectioners sugar substitute
- 3 tablespoons of freshly squeezed lemon juice
- 2 tablespoons of heavy whipping cream
- 1 teaspoon of lemon extract
- 2 teaspoons of lemon zest

Instructions

Keto Blueberry Lemon Bread

- Preheat oven to 350 degrees.
- Grease and line with parchment paper a 10X5 inch loaf pan or two 6 inch loaf pans. (note if using two smaller pans check for doneness at 35 minute mark)
- In a medium-sized bowl measure then sift the almond flour. To the sifted flour add the baking powder, sea salt and stir. Set this aside.
- In a large bowl using an electric hand-held mixer or stand-up mixer blend the butter, cream cheese, and sugar-substitute until mixture is light fluffy.
- Next add the 8 eggs one at a time, making sure to scrape the bowl several times.
- To the wet batter add the dry ingredients and combine until well-incorporated.
- Fold in the blueberries into the bread batter.
- Spread the batter into the greased loaf pan.
- Bake for 60-70 minutes or until an inserted toothpick comes out clean.
- Allow the loaf to cool in the pan for about 30 minutes before taking it out of the pan. Then let the pan cool on a baking rack for at least 60 minutes before adding the icing, refrigerating or freezing.

Keto Lemon Glaze

- To make the lemon glaze imply combine the confectioners sugar substitute, lemon juice, lemon extract, lemon zest and heavy whipping cream. Stir until fully incorporated.

Nutrition Info

Calories: 350 Total Fat: 30.6g Saturated Fat: 11.4g Cholesterol: 154mg
Sodium: 157mg Carbohydrates: 7.2g Fiber: 3.5g Sugar: 2.3g Protein: 10.3g

7 ULTIMATE DAIRY-FREE KETO BREAD

Prep Time 5 minutes
Cook Time 30 minutes
Servings 4

Ingredients

- 2 oz. macadamia butter OR 3.5 T almond butter + 0.5 T oil (2 oz. total)
- 2 large eggs
- 1 large egg white
- 1 oz. coconut flour
- 1/2 tsp. baking powder
- 1/4 tsp. salt
- 1/2 tsp. erythritol
- 1/2 tbsp. psyllium husks powder

Instructions

- Preheat the oven to 350°F (180°C). Line a baking pan with a sheet of parchment paper.
- In a small bowl, combine all the dry ingredients, leaving out only the psyllium husks powder. The coconut flour is best sifted.
- Ultimate Keto Bread
- Make macadamia butter if you don't have any. Just pulse the nuts in a bowl of an S-blade food processor (scraping the sides of the bowl once or twice) until you get runny
- butter. Ultimate Keto Bread
- Mix the eggs and the egg white in a medium bowl using an electric mixer. Add the macadamia butter and mix again until well incorporated.
- Ultimate Keto Bread
- Combine the egg mixture and the dry mixture, and mix well. At the very end, add the psyllium husks powder and mix some more. If you find the mixture to be runny, add in another T of coconut flour and mix well.
- Ultimate Keto Bread

- Use your hands or a spoon to form four disks on the baking pan. Wet your hands to make this step less sticky.
- Bake for 30 minutes.

Nutrition Info

170 Calories,
Fat: 13.4 g (of which Saturated: 3.4 g, MUFA's: 9.3 g),
Total Carbs: 7.5 g,
Fiber: 4.9 g,
Net Carbs: 2.6 g,
Protein: 6.5 g

---

8 COCONUT FLOUR PIZZA CRUST

This coconut flour pizza crust is the best gluten-free pizza crust I've ever tried. It's soft and tasty, and sturdy enough to hold with your hands!

Prep Time10 mins
Cook Time20 mins
Total Time30 mins
Servings: 2 (8-inch) pizzas

Ingredients

- Olive oil spray for pans
- 4 large eggs
- 2 tablespoons water
- 1 teaspoon garlic powder
- 1 teaspoon onion powder
- 1 teaspoon dried oregano
- 1/4 cup coconut flour
- 6 tablespoons grated parmesan cheese (1 oz)

Topping:

- 1/2 cup marinara sauce
- 1 cup shredded part-skim mozzarella (4 oz)

Instructions

- Preheat oven to 400 degrees F.
- Line two pizza pans with parchment paper and spray the paper with olive oil. You can also make these pizzas side by side on a single, large baking sheet.
- In a large bowl, whisk the eggs with the water, garlic powder, onion powder and dried oregano.
- Measure out the coconut flour, breaking up any lumps with your hands. Stir the coconut flour into the egg mixture, mixing until smooth.
- Stir in the Parmesan cheese.
- Allow the mixture to rest and thicken for a couple of minutes. This will allow the coconut flour to soak up the liquid.
- Using a rubber spatula, transfer half of the mixture onto each of the prepared pans. Use a spatula to spread it out evenly into an 8-inch circle.
- Bake the pizzas until set and the edges are beginning to brown, about 15 minutes. The crust will still be light at this point, and that's OK.
- Remove the pizzas from the oven and switch the oven to broil. Position the top oven rack 6 inches below flame.
- Spread each pizza with half the pizza sauce, sprinkle with half the shredded mozzarella, and add any other toppings you like (I used Applegate's pepperoni).
- Broil each pizza until cheese is melted and crust is golden-brown, 2-3 minutes.

Nutrition Info

Calories 496 Calories from Fat 297
Total Fat 33g 51%
Saturated Fat 15g 75%
Sodium 885mg 37%
Total Carbohydrates 13g 4%
Dietary Fiber 5g 20%
Sugars 14g

9 SWEET KETO CHALLAH BREAD RECIPE

Sweet Keto Challah Bread Recipe (Braided) is made into perfection without Flour, perfect for Low Carb option.

Prep Time 10 minutes
Cook Time 45 minutes
Total Time 55 minutes
20 Serving

Ingredients

- 4 Eggs
- 50g (1/3 Cup)Sukrin Plus
- 345g (1,5 Cup) Cream Cheese
- 60g (1/4 Cup)Butter
- 60g (1/4 Cup)Heavy Cream
- 50g (1/4 Cup)Oil
- 1 Cup (100g) Unflavored Protein
- 2/3 Cup (85g) Vanilla Protein
- 1/2 tsp salt
- 1/3 tsp (3g) Baking Soda
- 2 1/2 tsp (12g) Baking Powder
- 1 tsp (4g) Xanthan
- 1/2 of Lemon Zest
- 1/4 Cup (30g) Dried Berries (I have used cranberries)

Instructions

- Heat up the oven to 160C or 320F
- In a separate bowl, mix eggs into fluffiness, then add sugar substitute and mix again.
- Add Cream Cheese and all of the liquid ingredients and mix again
- Once that is properly mixed, add all of the dried ingredients and finish it with mixing it all together.
- Take it our of the mixer and add fresh lemon zest followed by dry cranberries
- Gently hand mix it into the dough, which is then poured into a

silicone baking pan, depending on your desired shape.

- Bake for 45 Min
- Bon appetite

Nutrition Info

Calories: 158
Total Fat: 13g
Saturated Fat: 6g
Trans Fat: 0g
Unsaturated Fat: 6g
Cholesterol: 66mg
Sodium: 241mg
Carbohydrates: 2g
Protein: 9g

10 Keto Cheddar Bay Biscuits

These keto cheddar bay biscuits taste so much like Red Lobster biscuits!

Try this copycat recipe for savory, cheesy, and EASY keto dinner rolls.

Prep time: 5 mins
Cook time: 25 mins
Total time: 30 mins

Ingredients:

- 2 cups almond flour (what we used)
- 2 teaspoons baking powder
- 1/2 teaspoon Himalayan salt
- 1/2 teaspoon garlic powder
- 1/4 teaspoon ground black pepper
- 4 tablespoons grass-fed unsalted butter, chilled and cut into small pieces
- 4 tablespoons heavy whipping cream
- 2 large eggs, beaten
- 4 ounces white cheddar cheese, shredded
- 2 ounces sharp yellow cheddar cheese, shredded
- 1 tablespoon dried parsley

Instructions

- Preheat oven to 350 degrees. Line a baking sheet with parchment or a silicone baking liner.
- In a large mixing bowl, blend all dry ingredients. Add butter and crumble with a fork (or your hands, if they're cold) until incorporated well into the dry mix.
- Add heavy cream in small amounts, mixing well between each addition. Stir eggs into the mixture. Mix white cheddar into the batter until it forms a doughy consistency, then gently add in yellow cheddar.
- Scoop 8 even portions of dough onto your prepared baking sheet. (You can also roll into balls instead if you want rounder biscuits.)
- Bake for 20 minutes, or until browned on the bottom.
- Serve warm, or cool completely and store in a covered container. Reheat gently in a toaster oven when ready to serve again.

Calories 350
Fat (grams) 32
Sat. Fat (grams) 12
Carbs (grams) 6.2

---

11 BUTTERY LOW CARB FLATBREAD

The best thing since sliced bread. Mostly because it's gluten-free, fried, and slathered in butter.

Prep time 5 mins
Cook time 2 mins
Total time 7 mins
Serves: 4

Ingredients

- 1 cup Almond Flour
- 2 tbsp Coconut Flour

- 2 tsp Xanthan Gum
- ½ tsp Baking Powder
- ½ tsp Falk Salt + more to garnish
- 1 Whole Egg + 1 Egg White
- 1 tbsp Water
- 1 tbsp Oil for frying
- 1 tbsp melted Butter-for slathering

Instructions

- Whisk together the dry ingredients (flours, xanthan gum, baking powder, salt) until well combined.
- Add the egg and egg white and beat gently into the flour to incorporate. The dough will begin to form.
- Add the tablespoon of water and begin to work the dough to allow the flour and xanthan gum to absorb the moisture.
- Cut the dough in 4 equal parts and press each section out with cling wrap. Watch the video for instructions!
- Heat a large skillet over medium heat and add oil.
- Fry each flatbread for about 1 min on each side.
- Brush with butter (while hot) and garnish with salt and chopped parsley.

Nutrition Info

Serving size: 1 flatbread Calories: 232 Fat: 19 Carbohydrates: 9 Fiber: 5 Protein: 9

12 THE BEST KETO DINNER ROLLS

These are the best keto dinner rolls to help replace bread in your low carb lifestyle. This recipe is easy, filling, and delicious!

Prep Time: 5 minutes
Cook Time: 10 minutes
Total Time: 15 minutes
Serving: 6 rolls

Ingredients

- 1 Cup Mozzarella, shredded
- 1 oz Cream Cheese
- 1 Cup Almond Flour
- 1/4 Cup Ground Flax Seed
- 1 egg
- 1/2 Tsp Baking Soda

Instructions

- Preheat oven to 400
- Line baking sheet with parchment, set aside
- In a medium bowl, melt cream cheese and mozzarella together (microwave ~1 min)
- Stir cheeses together until smooth, add egg and stir until combined
- In separate bowl combine almond flour, ground flax seed and baking soda
- Mix cheese and egg mixture into dry ingredients and stir until dough forms soft ball (it will be sticky)
- Using wet hands, gently roll dough into 6 balls
- Roll tops in sesame seeds if desired and place onto lined baking sheet
- Bake for 10-12 minutes until golden
- brown Let cool for 15 minutes

Nutrition Info

Serving Size: 1 roll
Calories: 219
Fat: 18g
Carbohydrates: 5.6g total (2.3g NET)
Fiber: 3.3g

Protein: 10.7g

---

13 NUT-FREE KETO BUNS

Hands-on 10-15 minutes
Overall 1 hour 15 minutes
Serving: 10 buns

Ingredients

Dry ingredients

- 1 1/4 cup fine defatted sesame seed flour (100 g / 3.5 oz)
- 2/3 cup flaxmeal (100 g / 3.5 oz)
- 2/3 cup coconut flour (80 g / 2.8 oz)
- 1/3 packed cup psyllium husk powder (40 g / 1.4 oz)
- 2 tsp garlic powder
- 2 tsp onion powder
- 2 tsp cream of tartar or apple cider vinegar
- 1 tsp baking soda
- 1 tsp salt (pink Himalayan or sea salt)
- 5 tbsp sesame seeds (or sunflower, flax, poppy seeds) or 1-2 tbsp caraway seeds for topping

Wet ingredients

- 6 large egg whites
- 2 large eggs
- 2 1/4 - 2 1/2 cups water depending on the consistency, boiling or lukewarm depending on the method - see intro (540 ml / 18 fl oz) - Use only 2 cups if using ground sesame seeds / sesame seed meal instead of defatted sesame seed flour.

Instructions

- Preheat the oven to 175 °C/ 350 °F. Use a kitchen scale to measure all the ingredients carefully. I used defatted sesame seed flour but you can try sesame seed meal instead and use less water. To make sesame seed meal, I just blend the seeds until powdered (just like I do with flax seeds to make flax meal).
- I used Sukrin sesame flour (UK) but you can use this brand too (US) - both should be defatted. Nut-Free Keto Buns
- Mix all the dry ingredients apart from the seeds for the topping in a bowl: sesame flour, coconut flour, flaxmeal, psyllium powder, ...
- Do not use whole psyllium husks - if you cannot find psyllium husk powder, use a blender or coffee grinder and process until fine. If you get already prepared psyllium husk powder, remember to weigh it before adding to the recipe. I used whole psyllium husks which I grinded myself. Do not use just measure cups - different products have different weights per cup! Nut-Free
- ..., baking soda, cream of tartar, garlic powder, ...
- Cream of tartar and baking soda act as leavening agents. This is how it works: To get 2 teaspoons of gluten-free baking powder, you need 1/2 a teaspoon of baking soda and 1 teaspoon of cream of tartar (double in this recipe of 10 buns). If you don't have cream of tartar, instead you can use apple cider vinegar and add it to the wet
- ingredients. Nut-Free Keto Buns ... onion powder and salt
- Add the egg whites and eggs and process well using a mixer until the dough is thick.
- Nut-Free Keto Buns The reason you shouldn't use only whole eggs is that the buns wouldn't rise with so many egg yolks in. Don't waste them - use them for making Home-made Mayo, Easy Hollandaise Sauce or Lemon Curd.
- Add boiling water and mix until well combined. Nut-Free Keto Buns
- Using a spoon or hands, form the buns and place them on a non-stick baking tray or a parchment paper. They will grow in

size as they bake, so make sure to leave some space between them. Top each of the buns with sesame seeds (or any other seeds) and press them into the dough, so they don't fall out.

- Place in the oven and cook for 55-60 minutes. Remove from the oven, let the tray cool down and place the buns on a rack to cool down to room temperature. Store them at room temperature if you plan to use them in the next couple of days or in the freezer for future use.
- Top with butter or cream cheese, burger meat and meat-free toppings. Enjoy!

Nutrition Info

Net carbs3.5 grams
Protein12.3 grams
Fat10.6 grams
Calories180 kcal

14 CAULIFLOWER BREAD RECIPE WITH GARLIC & HERBS - LOW CARB GARLIC BREAD

This cauliflower bread loaf with garlic & herbs makes a keto, paleo, low carb garlic bread that's healthy & delicious! Great for low carb sandwiches, too.

Prep Time 15 minutes
Cook Time 45 minutes
Total Time 1 hour

Ingredients

- 3 cup Cauliflower ("riced" using food processor*)
- 10 large Egg (separated)
- 1/4 tsp Cream of tartar (optional)

- 1 1/4 cup Coconut flour
- 1 1/2 tbsp Gluten-free baking powder
- 1 tsp Sea salt
- 6 tbsp Butter (unsalted, measured solid, then melted; can use ghee for dairy-free)
- 6 cloves Garlic (minced)
- 1 tbsp Fresh rosemary (chopped)
- 1 tbsp Fresh parsley (chopped)

Instructions

- Preheat the oven to 350 degrees F (177 degrees C). Line a 9x5 in (23x13 cm) loaf pan with parchment paper.
- Steam the riced cauliflower. You can do this in the microwave (cooked for 3-4 minutes, covered in plastic) OR in a steamer basket over water on the stove (line with cheesecloth if the holes in the steamer basket are too big, and steam for a few minutes). Both ways, steam until the cauliflower is soft and tender. Allow the cauliflower to cool enough to handle.
- Meanwhile, use a hand mixer to beat the egg whites and cream of tartar until stiff peaks form.
- Place the coconut flour, baking powder, sea salt, egg yolks, melted butter, garlic, and 1/4 of the whipped egg whites in a food processor.
- When the cauliflower has cooled enough to handle, wrap it in kitchen towel and squeeze several times to release as much moisture as possible. (This is important - the end result should be very dry and clump together.) Add the cauliflower to the food processor. Process until well combined. (Mixture will be dense and a little crumbly.)
- Add the remaining egg whites to the food processor. Fold in just a little, to make it easier to process. Pulse a few times until just incorporated. (Mixture will be fluffy.) Fold in the chopped parsley and rosemary. (Don't overmix to avoid breaking down the egg whites too much.)
- Transfer the batter into the lined baking pan. Smooth the top and round slightly. If desired, you can press more herbs into the

top (optional).

- Bake for about 45-50 minutes, until the top is golden. Cool completely before removing and slicing.
- How To Make Buttered Low Carb Garlic Bread (optional): Top slices generously with butter, minced garlic, fresh parsley, and a little sea salt. Bake in a preheated oven at 450 degrees F (233 degrees C) for about 10 minutes. If you want it more browned, place under the broiler for a couple of minutes.

Nutrition Info

Calories 108
Fat 8g
Protein 6g
Total Carbs 8g
Net Carbs 3g
Fiber 5g
Sugar 3g

---

15 PARMESAN & TOMATO KETO BREAD BUNS

Prep Time: 10-15 minutes
Total Time: 55-60 minutes

Ingredients

Dry ingredients:

- 3/4 cup almond flour (75 g/ 2.7 oz)
- 2 1/2 tbsp psyllium husk powder (20 g/ 0.7 oz)
- 1/4 cup coconut flour (30 g/ 1.1 oz)
- 1/4 cup packed cup flax meal (38 g/ 1.3
- oz) 1 tsp cream of tartar or apple cider
- vinegar 1/2 tsp baking soda
- 2/3 cup grated Parmesan cheese (60 g/ 2.1
- oz) 1/3 cup chopped sun-dried tomatoes (37
- g/ 1.3 oz) 1/4 - 1/2 tsp pink sea salt
- 2 tbsp sesame seeds (18 g/ 0.6 oz) - or use 2 tbsp sunflower,

flax, poppy seeds, or 1 tbsp caraway seeds

Wet ingredients:

- 3 large egg whites
- 1 large egg
- 1 cups boiling water (240 ml/ 8 fl oz)

Instructions

- Preheat the oven to 175 °C/ 350 °F (fan assisted). Use a kitchen scale to measure all the ingredients and add them to a mixing bowl (apart from the sesame seeds which are used for topping): almond flour, coconut flour, flax meal, psyllium husk powder, cream of tartar, baking soda, salt, parmesan cheese and sun dried tomatoes. Mix all the dry ingredients together. Parmesan & Tomato Keto Bread Buns
- Add the egg whites and eggs and process well using a mixer until the dough is thick.
- The reason you shouldn't use only whole eggs is that the buns wouldn't rise with so many egg yolks in. Don't waste them - use them for making Home-made Mayo, Easy Hollandaise Sauce or Lemon Curd. Parmesan & Tomato Keto Bread Buns
- Add boiling water and process until well combined. Parmesan & Tomato Keto Bread Buns
- Using a spoon, divide the keto buns mix into 5 and roll into buns using your hands. Place them on a non-stick baking tray or on parchment paper. They will grow in size, so make sure to leave some space between them. You can even use small tart trays.
- Top each of the buns with sesame seeds (or any other seeds) and gently press them into the dough, so they don't fall out. Place in the oven and cook for about 45 - 50 minutes until golden on top. Parmesan & Tomato Keto Bread Buns
- Remove from the oven, let the tray cool down and place the buns on a rack to cool to room temperature. Parmesan & Tomato Keto Bread Buns
- Enjoy just like you would regular bread — with butter, ham or

cheese! Parmesan & Tomato Keto Bread Buns Store in a tupperware for 2-3 days or freeze for up to 3 months.

Nutrition Info

Calories261 kcal
Net carbs4.9 grams
Protein14.5 grams
Fat18.9 grams

16 COCONUT BREAD

Prep/Cook Time: 60 mins

Ingredients

- 1/2 cup coconut flour
- 1/4 tsp salt
- 1/4 tsp baking soda
- 6 eggs
- ¼ cup coconut oil, melted
- ¼ unsweetened almond milk

Instructions

- Preheat oven to 350°F.
- Line an 8×4 inch loaf pan with parchment paper.
- In a bowl combine the coconut flour, baking soda and salt.
- In another bowl combine the eggs, milk and oil.
- Slowly add the wet ingredients into the dry ingredients and mix until combined.
- Pour the mixture into the prepared loaf pan.
- Bake for 40-50 minutes, or until a toothpick, inserted in the middle comes out clean.

Nutrition Info

Calories 108
Carbohydrates 3.4 g
Fat 8.7 g
Potassium 35.8 mg
Folic Acid (B9) 12.1 μg
Sodium 86 mg

17 KETO CREAM CHEESE BREAD

Prep Time: 5 minutes
Cook Time: 25 minutes
Additional Time: 5 minutes
Total Time: 35 minutes
Serving: 12

Ingredients

- 8 large eggs
- 8 ounces of full-fat cream cheese (room temperature)
- ½ cup of unsalted butter (room temperature)
- 1 ½ cups coconut flour
- ½ cup of full-fat sour cream
- 4 teaspoons of baking powder
- 1 teaspoon of sea salt
- 1 tablespoon of sugar substitute

- 2 tablespoons of sesame seeds (optional)

Instructions

- Allow your eggs, cream cheese, butter to come to room temperature.
- Pre-heat your oven to 350 degrees.
- Grease a 12 cavity muffin pan generously with butter or a 10 inch loaf pan.
- In a medium-sized bowl combine your coconut flour, baking powder, sea salt, sugar substitute and set aside.
- In a large bowl using a handheld electric mixer or a standup mixer beat together the room temperature butter, cream cheese until light and fluffy. Be sure to scrape the sides of bowl several times to make sure the mixture is well blended.
- To this butter and cream cheese mixture add the 8 eggs one at a time. Making sure to scrape the sides of the bowl several times. Note that due to the large number of eggs the mixture will not fully combine, this is normal. Once you add the dry ingredients to this wet mixture, the ingredients will come together perfectly.
- To the wet ingredients slowly add all the dry ingredients on a low mixing setting. Making sure to scrape the bowl a couple of times.
- Once the two mixtures are fully combined stop using the electric mixture and fold in the 1/2 cup of sour cream gently. Making sure the sour cream gets fully incorporated into the batter but being careful to not over mix.Note that the batter will be very thick and fluffy. This is the normal texture when using coconut flour exclusively in a recipe.
- Overfill the muffin pan just slightly. The thick batter will not cause the muffins to spread. Slightly overfilling your muffin tins will create a nice muffin top.
- With one additional whole egg and a tablespoon of water create an egg wash. Baste the top of each muffin with the egg wash and then sprinkle the sesame seeds on top of each muffin. This step is optional.
- Bake the muffins for 25-30 minutes until lightly brown on the

top and when an inserted toothpick comes out clean.

- Report this ad
- If you are baking your keto cream cheese bread in a 10 inch loaf, bake the bread for up to 90 minutes. Check your bread at 60 minutes for doneness and allow to cook longer if necessary.

Nutrition Info

Calories: 204 Total Fat: 19.4g Saturated Fat: 11.4g Cholesterol: 154mg Sodium: 160mg Carbohydrates: 2.2g Fiber: 0.6g Sugar: 0.4g Protein: 5.8g

---

18 KETO BANANA BREAD

Prep Time: 10 minutes
Cook Time: 1 hour
Total Time: 1 hour 5 minutes
Servings: 16 serves

Ingredients

- 80 g butter melted
- 25 g sugar free maple syrup
- 1 cup (150g) Sukrin Gold sweetener or Lakanto Gold sweetener
- 2 teaspoons ground cinnamon
- 1/2 teaspoon nutmeg fresh grated
- 1 teaspoon vanilla
- 100 g banana
- 60 g golden flax meal or golden flax seeds milled extra fine
- 20 g coconut flour
- 150 g almond meal
- 1 tablespoon baking powder I totally recommend Bobs Red Mill Baking Powder for best rise
- 10 g psyllium husk powder or chia flour

- 1 teaspoon xanthan gum
- 4 eggs
- 80 g Greek natural yogurt

OPTIONAL

- 2 teaspoons banana extract INSTEAD of banana
- 1 cup walnuts or brazil nuts chopped

Instructions

- Preheat oven 170?. Line a 22cm x 11cm loaf tine with baking paper.

Conventional Method

- Over medium heat cook butter, maple syrup, sweetener, cinnamon and nutmeg until butter has melted.
- In a large mixing bowl mash bananas. Pour in melted butter mixture and combine well.
- Add remaining ingredients including nuts (if using) and fold until combined.
- Scoop batter into prepared loaf tin. Smooth over top of loaf with wet spatula.
- Bake 60 minutes or until a skewer comes out clean. Cool 5 minutes in pan before transferring to wire rack to cool completely.

Thermomix Method

- Add butter, maple syrup, sweetener, cinnamon and nutmeg and cook 5 minutes/100?/stir.
- Add banana and mix 10 seconds speed 4. Scrape sides of bowl
- Add remaining ingredients. Mix 30 seconds/speed 3. Fold though nuts (if using) Follow instructions from Step 4 above.

Nutrition Info

Calories: 141kcal, Carbohydrates: 6g, Protein: 4g, Fat: 11g, Saturated Fat: 3g, Cholesterol: 51mg, Sodium: 63mg, Potassium: 150mg, Fiber: 2g, Sugar: 1g, Vitamin A: 3.8%, Vitamin C: 0.7%, Calcium: 7.7%, Iron: 5%

---

19 CRANBERRY JALAPEÑO "CORNBREAD" MUFFINS

Low carb, grain-free muffins that taste like cornbread! Made with coconut flour and bursting with cranberries and jalapeño, these delicious muffins would make a great addition to any Thanksgiving table.

Prep Time 10 mins
Cook Time 30 mins
Total Time 40 mins
Servings: 12 muffins
Calories: 157 kcal

Ingredients

- 1 cup coconut flour (I used Bob's Red Mill)
- 1/3 cup Swerve Sweetener or other erythritol
- 1 tbsp baking powder
- 1/2 tsp salt
- 7 large eggs, lightly beaten
- 1 cup unsweetened almond milk
- 1/2 cup butter, melted OR avocado oil
- 1/2 tsp vanilla
- 1 cup fresh cranberries, cut in half
- 3 tbsp minced jalapeño peppers
- 1 jalapeño, seeds removed, sliced into 12 slices, for garnish

Instructions

- Preheat oven to 325F and grease a muffin tin well or line with paper liners.
- In a medium bowl, whisk together coconut flour, sweetener, baking powder and salt. Break up any clumps with the back of a fork.
- Stir in eggs, melted butter and almond milk and stir vigorously. Stir in vanilla extract and continue to stir until mixture is smooth and well combined. Stir in chopped cranberries and jalapeños.
- Divide batter evenly among prepared muffin cups and place one slice of jalapeño on top of each.
- Bake 25 to 30 minutes or until tops are set and a tester inserted in the center comes out clean. Let cool 10 minutes in pan, then transfer to a wire rack to cool completely.

Nutrition Info

Calories 157 Calories from Fat 101
Total Fat 11.22g 17%
Dietary Fiber 3.84g 15%
Protein 5.21g 10%

---

20 LOW CARB PUMPKIN BREAD

Prep Time: 15 minutes
Cook Time: 45 minutes
Total Time: 1 hour
Serving: 20

Ingredients

- 15 oz. can of pumpkin puree
- 2 cups granulated of sugar substitute
- 3 teaspoons of baking powder
- 2 teaspoon vanilla extract
- 3 tablespoons of pumpkin pie spice
- 3 tablespoons of cinnamon powder
- 1/4 teaspoon sea salt

- 10 large eggs
- 3 cups of almond flour
- 1 cup of golden flax meal
- Optional
- Cream Cheese Frosting
- 8 oz package of softened cream cheese
- 4 tablespoons of heavy whipping cream
- 1 cup of sugar-free confectioners sugar

Instructions

- Preheat oven to 350 degrees.
- Grease two 8x4 inch loaf pans well.
- Using an electric mixer, beat the pumpkin puree, sugar substitute, and vanilla extract until well blended.
- Next add in the eggs one at time making sure to beat until fully combined.
- To the wet batter add the almond flour, flax meal, baking powder, spices and salt.
- Note that batter will be thick. Pour the batter into the two prepared pans and bake at 350 degrees for 45 minutes, or until an inserted toothpick comes out clean.

Nutrition Info

Calories: 200 Total Fat: 15.8g Saturated Fat: 5.5g Cholesterol: 59mg Sodium: 60mg Carbohydrates: 4.8g Fiber: 2.9g Sugar: 0.8g Protein: 6.4g

21 COCONUT FLOUR FLATBREAD

Coconut flour flatbread Ketogenic flatbread perfect as a side to curries or a low carb tortillas wraps. 100% Vegan + eggless + gluten free soft breads.

Prep Time10 mins
Cook Time5 mins
Total Time15 mins
Servings: 6 flatbreads

Ingredients

- 2 tablespoons psyllium husk (9g)
- 1/2 cup coconut flour fine, fresh, no lumps (60g)
- 1 cup lukewarm water (240ml)
- 1 tablespoon olive oil (15ml)
- 1/4 teaspoons baking soda
- 1/4 teaspoons salt - optional

Cooking

- 1 teaspoon olive oil to rub/oil the non stick pan

Instructions

Make the dough

- In a medium mixing bowl, combine the psyllium husk and coconut flour (if lumps are in your flour use a fork to smash them BEFORE measuring the flour, amount must be precise).
- Add in the lukewarm water (I used tap water about 40C/bath temperature), olive oil, and baking soda. Give a good stir with a spatula, then use your hands to knead the dough. Add salt now if you want. I never add the salt in contact with baking soda to avoid deactivating the leaving agent.
- Knead for 1 minute. The dough is moist and it gets softer and slightly dryer as you go. It should come together easily to form a dough as on my picture. If not, too sticky, add more husk, 1/2 teaspoon at a time, knead for 30 sec and see how it goes. The dough will always be a bit moist but it shouldn't stick to your hands at all. It must come together as a dough.

- Set aside 10 minute in the mixing bowl.
- Now the dough must be soft, elastic and hold well together, it is ready to roll.

Roll/ shape the flatbread

- Cut the dough into 4 even pieces, roll each pieces into a small ball.
- Place one of the dough ball between two pieces of parchment paper, press the ball with your hand palm to stick it well to the paper and start rolling with a rolling pin as thin as you like a bread. My breads are 20 cm diameter (8 inches) and I made 6 flatbread with this recipe.
- Un peel the first layer of parchment paper from your flatbread. Use a lid to cut out round flatbread. Keep the outside dough to reform a ball and roll more flatbread - that is how I make 2 extra flatbread from the 4 balls above!

Nutrition Info

Serving: 1flatbread, Calories: 66kcal, Carbohydrates: 7.3g, Protein: 2g, Fat: 3.3g, Fiber: 4.7g, Sugar: 2g

22 LOW CARB BLUEBERRY ENGLISH MUFFIN BREAD LOAF

Prep Time 15 minutes
Cook Time 45 minutes
Total Time 1 hour
Servings 12

Ingredients

- 1/2 cup almond butter or cashew or peanut butter

- 1/4 cup butter ghee or coconut oil
- 1/2 cup almond flour
- 1/2 tsp salt
- 2 tsp baking powder
- 1/2 cup almond milk unsweetened
- 5 eggs beaten
- 1/2 cup blueberries

Instructions

- Preheat oven to 350 degrees F.

- In a microwavable bowl melt nut butter and butter together for 30 seconds, stir until combined well.

- In a large bowl, whisk almond flour, salt and baking powder together. Pour the nut butter mixture into the large bowl and stir to combine.
- Whisk the almond milk and eggs together then pour into the bowl and stir well.

- Drop in fresh blueberries or break apart frozen blueberries and gently stir into the batter.
- Line a loaf pan with parchment paper and lightly grease the parchment paper as well.
- Pour the batter into the loaf pan and bake 45 minutes or until a toothpick in center comes out clean.
- Cool for about 30 minutes then remove from pan.

- Slice and toast each slice before serving.

DOUGH

The BEST recipe for cheesy keto garlic bread - using mozzarella dough. At only 1.5g net carbs per slice, this is an absolute keeper for your low-carb recipe folder.

Prep Time10 mins
Cook Time15 mins
Total Time25 mins
Servings: 10

Ingredients

- 170 g pre shredded/grated cheese mozzarella
- 85 g almond meal/flour
- 2 tbsp cream cheese full fat
- 1 tbsp garlic crushed
- 1 tbsp parsley fresh or dried
- 1 tsp baking powder
- pinch salt to taste
- 1 egg medium

Instructions

- Place all the ingredients apart from the egg, in a microwaveable bowl. Stir gently to mix together. Microwave on HIGH for 1 minute.
- Stir then microwave on HIGH for a further 30 seconds.
- Add the egg then mix gently to make a cheesy dough.
- Place on a baking tray and form into a garlic bread shape. Cut slices into the low-carb garlic bread.
- Optional: Mix 2 tbsp melted butter, 1 tsp parsley and 1 tsp garlic. Brush over the top of the low-carb garlic bread, sprinkle with more cheese.
- Bake at 220C/425F for 15 minutes, or until golden brown.

Nutrition Info

Calories 117.4 Calories from Fat 88
Total Fat 9.8g 15%
Total Carbohydrates 2.4g 1%
Dietary Fiber 0.9g 4%
Sugars 0.6g
Protein 6.2g 12%

---

24 CINNAMON RAISIN SWIRL BREAD

A low carb Cinnamon Raisin Swirl Bread that does the original justice! Enjoy this naturally sweet and healthy treat for your holiday brunch or breakfast.

Prep Time 20 mins
Cook Time 1 hr 10 mins
Total Time 1 hr 30 mins
Servings: 1 loaf

Ingredients

Filling:

- 1 tbsp Swerve Sweetener
- 1 tsp ground cinnamon

Bread:

- 1/2 cup coconut flour
- 1/2 cup almond flour
- 6 tbsp psyllium husk powder
- 1/4 cup California raisins chopped fine
- 2 tbsp Swerve Sweetener
- 1 tbsp baking powder
- 1/2 tsp ground cinnamon
- 1/4 tsp salt
- 2 cups egg whites (liquid egg whites work well but you can also measure out whites from regular eggs. It will be 8 to 12 whites, depending on the size)

- 4 tbsp melted butter divided
- 2 tbsp apple cider vinegar
- 3/4 cup hot water (almost boiling)

Instructions

- Preheat oven to 350F and grease a 9x5 inch loaf pan. Grease 2 large pieces of parchment paper.
- In a small bowl, whisk together the sweetener and cinnamon. Set aside.
- In a large bowl, whisk together the coconut flour, almond flour, psyllium husk powder, chopped raisins, sweetener, baking powder, cinnamon and salt.
- Add egg whites, 3 tbsp of the melted butter and the apple cider vinegar. Stir to combine. Slowly stir in hot water until dough expands.
- Turn dough out onto one of the pieces of greased parchment and pat into a rough rectangle. Top with other piece of parchment and roll out to about 8x 12 inches. Brush with about half of the remaining melted butter and sprinkle with cinnamon filling. Roll up tightly and place seam-side-down in prepared loaf pan.
- Brush with remaining butter. Bake 60 to 70 minutes, until golden brown and firm to the touch. Remove from oven and tent with foil. Let cool in pan (this will help keep it from deflating). Once cool, transfer it to a cutting board or serving plate.

Nutrition Info

Calories 132 Calories from Fat 59
Total Fat 6.58g 10%
Dietary Fiber 6.02g 24%
Protein 6.28g 13%

25 GRAIN FREE IRISH SODA BREAD (LOW CARB AND SUGAR-FREE)

Prep Time 15 minutes
Cook Time 40 minutes
Total Time 55 minutes
Servings 12 servings

Ingredients

- 2 cups sunflower seeds
- 1/2 cup ground flaxseed
- 2 tablespoons coconut flour
- 1/4 cup Swerve sweetener
- 2 teaspoon baking powder
- 1/2 teaspoon salt
- 2 tablespoons butter cold unsalted
- 2 eggs
- 1/4 cup coconut milk
- 1/4 cup raisins or currants

Instructions

- Preheat oven to 350 degrees.
- Grind the sunflower seeds in a food processor.
- Add the flaxseed, coconut flour, swerve, baking powder (or soda) and salt.
- Pulse in the butter.
- Add remaining ingredients, except raisins.
- Remove dough and transfer to a bowl.
- Mix in raisins or currants.
- Wet hands to form shape and place in a greased cast iron skillet.
- Score an x in the middle and bake 30 minutes.
- Reduce the temperature to 325 and bake another 5-10 minutes or until golden on top.
- Allow to cool before slicing.

26 KETO PULL APART CLOVER ROLLS

Prep Time 7 mins
Cook Time 20 mins
Total Time 27 mins
Servings:4

Ingredients

- 1 ½ cup blanched almond flour or can also use 1/3 cup coconut flour instead
- 1 ½ tsp baking powder
- 1 ½ cup shredded Mozzarella cheese
- 2 ounces cream cheese
- ¼ cup grated Parmesan cheese
- 2 lg eggs

Instructions

- Grease or spray with non-stick oil spray a muffin pan and preheat oven to 350 F.
- In a mixing bowl combine the almond flour and the baking powder, mix well. Set aside.
- Melt the shredded Mozzarella and the cream cheese on the stove top (or in the microwave for 1 minute) until melted.
- Once the cheese has melted, add flour mix, and eggs. Mix together.
- Grease hands and knead dough to form a sticky ball. Place the dough ball on a large sheet of baking paper or
- a silicon mat. Slice the dough ball into fourths. Then slice each quarter into 6 small pieces.
- Roll the small pieces into balls, and lightly roll the balls in a bowl of the Parmesan cheese to lightly coat them with Parmesan (this helps them be able to pull apart easily).
- Add 3 of the dough balls to each muffin cup in the muffin pan (this makes the 3 leaf clover).
- Bake at 350 F for 20 minutes or until golden brown. Remove from oven and allow to cool slightly before serving.

Nutrition Info

Calories 283 Calories from Fat 189
Total Fat 21g 32%
Saturated Fat 8g 40%
Total Carbohydrates 6g 2%
Dietary Fiber 2g 8%
Sugars 1g
Protein 16g 32%

---

27 SOUL BREAD SESAME ROLLS

Prep Time 15 mins
Cook Time 35 mins
Total Time 50 mins
Servings: 12 small rolls

Ingredients

- 8 ounces cream cheese softened
- 3 tbsp butter melted
- 2 1/2 tbsp avocado oil
- 2 1/2 tbsp whipping cream
- 2 eggs
- 1 egg white
- 1 cup plus 3 tbsp unflavoured whey protein powder
- 1 1/2 tsp baking powder
- 1/2 tsp xanthan gum
- 1/2 tsp garlic powder
- 1/4 plus 1/8 tsp salt
- 1/4 tsp baking soda
- 1/4 tsp cream of tartar
- Toasted sesame seeds

Instructions

- Preheat oven to 325F and grease a muffin top pan or a square brownie pan very well. You can also use a muffin pan.
- In a large bowl, beat together cream cheese, butter, avocado oil, whipping cream, eggs, and egg white.
- In another bowl, whisk together the protein powder, baking powder, xanthan gum, garlic powder, salt, baking soda, and cream of tartar. Break up any clumps with a fork.
- Add dry ingredients to the cream cheese mixture and fold in by hand until just combined. Do not over mix.
- Fill the cavities of prepared pan to almost full (for the muffin top pan, you may need to work in batches). Sprinkle tops with toasted sesame seeds.
- Bake 25 to 35 minutes, until golden brown on top and firm to the touch. Remove and let cool in pan 15 minutes, then flip out onto a wire rack to cool completely. *If using a muffin top pan, they won't take as long to bake. Keep your eye on them!

Nutrition Info

Calories 175 Calories from Fat 130
Total Fat 14.42g 22%
Cholesterol 67mg 22%
Total Carbohydrates 2.5g 1%
Dietary Fiber 0.33g 1%
Protein 9.34g 19%

28 GARLIC & HERB FOCACCIA {GRAIN FREE & LOW CARB}

Quit bread for good and get this grain free focaccia on your plate.

Prep time 10 mins
Cook time 20 mins
Total time 30 mins
Serves: 8 slices

Ingredients

Dry Ingredients

- 1 cup Almond Flour
- ¼ cup Coconut Flour
- ½ tsp Xanthan Gum
- 1 tsp Garlic Powder
- 1 tsp Flaky Salt
- ½ tsp Baking Soda
- ½ tsp Baking Powder

Wet Ingredients

- 2 eggs
- 1 tbsp Lemon Juice
- 2 tsp Olive oil + 2 tbsp Olive Oil to drizzle

Top with Italian Seasoning and TONS of flaky salt!

Instructions

- Heat oven to 350 and line a baking tray or 8-inch round pan with parchment.
- Whisk together the dry ingredients making sure there are no lumps.
- Beat the egg, lemon juice, and oil until combined.
- Mix the wet and the dry together, working quickly, and scoop the dough into your pan.
- **Make sure not to mix the wet and dry until you are ready to

put the bread in the oven because the leavening reaction begins once it is mixed!!!

- Smooth the top and edges with a spatula dipped in water (or your hands) then use your finger to dimple the dough. Don't be afraid to go deep on the dimples! Again, a little water keeps it from sticking.
- Bake covered for about 10 minutes. Drizzle with Olive Oil bake for an additional 10-15 minutes uncovering to brown gently.
- Top with more flaky salt, olive oil (optional), a dash of Italian seasoning and fresh basil. Let cool completely before slicing for optimal texture!!

Nutrition Info

Serving size: 1 Calories: 166 Fat: 13 Carbohydrates: 7 Fiber: 4 Protein: 7

---

29 KETO BAGEL RECIPE

Missing a good bagel in your Keto lifestyle? Now you don't have to!

Prep Time: 5 minutes
Cook Time: 25 minutes
Serving: 2

Ingredients

- 1 cup (120 g) of almond flour
- 1/4 cup (28 g) of coconut flour
- 1 Tablespoon (7 g) of psyllium husk powder
- 1 teaspoon (2 g) of baking powder
- 1 teaspoon (3 g) of garlic powder
- pinch salt
- 2 medium eggs (88 g)
- 2 teaspoons (10 ml) of white wine vinegar
- 2 1/2 Tablespoons (38 ml) of ghee, melted
- 1 Tablespoon (15 ml) of olive oil
- 1 teaspoon (5 g) of sesame seeds

Instructions

- Preheat the oven to 320°F (160°C).
- Combine the almond flour, coconut flour, psyllium husk powder, baking powder, garlic powder and salt in a bowl.
- In a separate bowl, whisk the eggs and vinegar together. Slowly drizzle in the melted ghee (which should not be piping hot) and whisk in well.
- Add the wet mixture to the dry mixture and use a wooden spoon to combine well. Leave to sit for 2-3 minutes.
- Divide the mixture into 4 equal-sized portions. Using your hands, shape the mixture into a round shape and place onto a tray lined with parchment paper. Use a small spoon or apple corer to make the center hole.
- Brush the tops with olive oil and scatter over the sesame seeds. Bake in the oven for 20-25 minutes until cooked through. Allow to cool slightly before enjoying!

Nutrition Info

Calories: 629 Sugar: 4 g Fat: 56 g Carbohydrates: 19 g Fiber: 12 g Protein: 19 g

---

30 KETO ZUCCHINI BREAD WITH WALNUTS

Servings: 4

Ingredients

- 3 large eggs
- ½ cup olive oil
- 1 teaspoon vanilla extract
- 2 ½ cups almond flour
- 1 ½ cups erythritol
- ½ teaspoon salt
- 1 ½ teaspoons baking powder
- ½ teaspoon nutmeg
- 1 teaspoon ground cinnamon

- ¼ teaspoon ground ginger
- 1 cup grated zucchini
- ½ cup chopped walnuts

Instructions

- Preheat oven to 350°F. Whisk together the eggs, oil, and vanilla extract. Set to the side.
- In another bowl, mix together the almond flour, erythritol, salt, baking powder, nutmeg, cinnamon, and ginger. Set to
- the side. Using a cheesecloth or paper towel, take the zucchini and squeeze out the excess water.
- Then, whisk the zucchini into the bowl with the eggs.
- Slowly add the dry ingredients into the egg mixture using a hand mixer until fully blended.
- Lightly spray a 9×5 loaf pan, and spoon in the zucchini bread mixture.
- Then, spoon in the chopped walnuts on top of the zucchini bread. Press walnuts into the batter using a spatula.
- Bake for 60-70 minutes at 350ºF or until the walnuts on top look browned.

Nutrition Info

200.13 Calories, 18.83g Fats, 2.6g Net Carbs, and 5.59g Protein.

31 PALEO GLUTEN-FREE LOW CARB ENGLISH MUFFIN RECIPE IN A MINUTE

A paleo low carb English muffin recipe that's soft and buttery inside, crusty on the outside. These gluten-free English muffins are easy to make in 2 minutes, with 5 ingredients!

Prep Time 2 minutes
Cook Time 3 minutes
Total Time 5 minutes

Ingredients

- 3 tbsp Blanched almond flour
- 1/2 tbsp Coconut flour
- 1 tbsp Butter (or ghee, or coconut oil)
- 1 large Egg (or equivalent egg whites)
- 1 pinch Sea salt
- 1/2 tsp Gluten-free baking powder

Instructions

- Melt ghee (or butter) in a microwave or oven safe ramekin or other container, about 4 in (10 cm) diameter with a flat bottom. This takes about 30 seconds. (If using the oven only, you can melt it in the oven while it preheats. Remove once melted.)
- Add the remaining ingredients and stir until well combined. Let sit for a minute to allow the mixture to thicken.
- Microwave method: Microwave for about 90 seconds, until firm.
- Oven method: Bake for about 15 minutes at 350 degrees F (177 degrees C), until the top is firm and spring-y to the touch.
- Run a knife along the edge and flip over a plate to release. Slice in half, then toast in the toaster.

Recipe Notes

- For more container options, see the list right above the recipe card (scroll up).
- If you prefer more/smaller slices, you can also make it in a mug instead of a ramekin, then just pop those in the toaster in batches.

Nutrition Info

Calories 307
Fat 27g
Protein 12g
Total Carbs 8g
Net Carbs 4g
Fiber 4g
Sugar 2g

---

32 CINNAMON ALMOND FLOUR BREAD {PALEO}

Prep Time: 10
Cook Time: 30 minutes
Total Time: 40 minutes
Serving: 8

Ingredients

- 2 cups fine blanched almond flour? (I use Bob's Red Mill)
- 2 tbsp coconut flour
- 1/2 tsp sea salt
- 1 tsp baking soda
- 1/4 cup Flax seed meal or chia meal ?(ground chia or flaxseed, see notes for how to make your own)
- 5 Eggs and 1 egg white whisked ??together
- 1.5 tsp Apple cider vinegar or lemon juice
- 2 tbsp maple syrup or honey
- 2–3 tbsp of clarified butter (melted) or Coconut oil; divided. Vegan butter also works
- 1 tbsp cinnamon plus extra for topping
- Optional chia seed to sprinkle of top before baking

Instructions

- Preheat oven to 350F. Line an 8×4 bread pan with parchment paper at the bottom and grease the sides.
- In a large bowl, mix together your almond flour, coconut flour, salt, baking soda, flaxseed meal or chia meal, and 1/2 tablespoon of cinnamon.

- In another small bowl, whisk together your eggs and egg white. Then add in your maple syrup (or honey), apple cider vinegar, and melted butter (1.5 to 2 tbsp).
- Mix wet ingredients into dry. Be sure to remove any clumps that might have occurred from the almond flour or coconut flour.
- Pour batter into a your greased loaf pan.
- Bake at 350º for 30-35 minutes, until a toothpick inserted into center of loaf comes out clean. Mine too around 35 minutes but I am at altitude.
- Remove from and oven.
- Next, whisk together the other 1 to 2 tbsp of melted butter (or oil) and mix it with 1/2 tbsp of cinnamon. Brush this on top of your cinnamon almond flour bread. Cool and serve
- or store for later.

Notes

- For storage, it's best to keep wrapped in foil or ziplock in fridge. The bread freezes well for meal prep.
- If you you use a larger pan, the loaf slices will be less fluffy but equally delicious.
- To make the flaxseed or chia meal, simply place the the flaxseeds or chia seeds in a coffee grinder and grind until a fine meal is formed.

Nutrition Info

Serving Size: 1
Calories Per Serving: 221
24% Total Fat 15.4g
13% Dietary Fiber 3.1g
Sugars 3.7g
19% Protein 9.3g
0% Vitamin C 0mg
9% Iron 1.5mg

33 GLUTEN FREE, PALEO & KETO BREAD

Prep Time: 15 minutes
Cook Time: 30 minutes
Resting Time: 40 minutes
Total Time: 45 minutes
Servings: 1

Ingredients

For the paleo & keto bread

- 2 teaspoons active dry yeast
- 2 teaspoons maple syrup or honey, to feed the yeast (NO SUGAR WILL BE REMAIN POST BAKE)
- 120 ml water lukewarm between 105-110°F
- 168 g almond flour
- 83 g golden flaxseed meal finely ground
- 15 g whey protein isolate
- 18 g psyllium husk finely ground
- 2 teaspoons xanthan gum or 4 teaspoons ground flaxseed meal**
- 2 teaspoons baking powder
- 1 teaspoon kosher salt
- 1/4 teaspoon cream of tartar
- 1/4 teaspoon ground ginger
- 1 egg at room temperature
- 110 g egg whites about 3, at room temperature
- 56 g grass-fed butter or ghee, melted and cooled
- 1 tablespoon apple cider vinegar
- 58 g sour cream or coconut cream + 2 tsp apple cider vinegar

Instructions

For the paleo & keto bread

- Line a 8.5 x 4.5 inch loaf pan with parchment paper (an absolute must!). Set aside.

- Add yeast and maple syrup (to feed the yeast, see notes) to a large bowl. Heat up water to 105-110°F, and if you don't have a thermometer it should only feel lightly warm to touch. Pour water over yeast mixture, cover bowl with a kitchen towel and allow to rest for 7 minutes. The mixture should be bubbly, if it isn't start again (too cold water won't activate the yeast and too hot will kill it).

- Mix your flours while the yeast is proofing. Add almond flour, flaxseed meal, whey protein powder, psyllium husk, xanthan gum, baking powder, salt, cream of tartar and ginger to a medium bowl and whisk until thoroughly mixed. Set aside.

- Once your yeast is proofed, add in the egg, egg whites, lightly cooled melted butter (you don't want to scramble the eggs or kill the yeast!) and vinegar. Mix with an electric mixer for a couple minutes until light and frothy. Add the flour mixture in two batches, alternating with the sour cream, and mixing until thoroughly incorporated. You want to mix thoroughly and q uickly to activate the xanthan gum, though the dough will become thick as the flours absorb the moisture.

- Transfer bread dough to prepared loaf pan, using a wet spatula to even out the top. Cover with a kitchen towel and place in a warm draft-free space for 50-60 minutes until the dough has risen just past the top of the loaf pan. How long it takes depends on your altitude, temperature and humidity- so keep an eye out for it every 15 minutes or so. And keep in mind that if you use a larger loaf pan it won't rise past the top.

- Preheat oven to 350°F/180°C while the dough is proofing. And if you're baking at high altitude, you'll want to bake it at 375°F/190°C.

- Place the loaf pan over a baking tray and transfer gently into the oven. Bake for 45-55 minutes until deep golden, covering with a lose foil dome at minute 10-15 (just as it begins to brown). Just be sure that the foil isn't resting directly on the bread.

- Allow the bread to rest in the loaf pan for 5 minutes and transfer it to a cooling rack. Allow to cool completely for best texture- this is an absolute must, as your keto loaf will continue to cook while cooling! Also keep in mind that some slight deflating is normal, don't sweat it!

- Keep stored in an airtight container (or tightly wrapped in cling film) at room temperature for 4-5 days, giving it a light toast before serving. Though you'll find that this keto bread is surprisingly good even without toasting!

Nutrition Info

Calories 174 Calories from Fat 126
Total Fat 14g 22%
Saturated Fat 3g 15%
Dietary Fiber 4g 16%
Protein 5g 10%

34 ALMOND FLOUR BREAD

An easy recipe for a quick, filling and tasty almond flour bread. This almond flour bread is keto and paleo, and works great with both savory and sweet toppings.

Prep Time10 mins
Cook Time45 mins
Rest time30 mins
Total Time1 hr 25 mins
Servings: 16 slices

Ingredients

- 1 teaspoon coconut oil for pan
- 5 large eggs
- 5 tablespoons refined coconut oil, gently melted in microwave (2.5 oz)

- 1 teaspoon apple cider vinegar (don't skip – helps the bread rise)
- 1/4 teaspoon kosher salt
- 1 3/4 cup almond flour (7 oz)
- 1/2 teaspoon baking soda

Instructions

- Preheat oven to 350 degrees F. Grease an 8-inch loaf pan (a 9-inch pan will be too big).
- In a medium bowl, whisk the eggs. Whisk in the coconut oil, vinegar, salt, almond flour and finally the baking soda.
- Pour the batter into the prepared loaf pan.
- Bake until bread is golden-brown and set, and a toothpick inserted in center comes out clean, about 45 minutes.
- Cool 10 minutes in pan on a wire rack before gently releasing the bread from the pan (carefully run a knife along edges if needed). Cool to room temperature, about 20 minutes more, before slicing and serving.
- Keep leftovers in a ziploc bag in the fridge for a few days, or freeze.

Nutrition Info

Calories 131 Calories from Fat 108
Total Fat 12g 18%
Sodium 83mg 3%
Total Carbohydrates 3g 1%
Dietary Fiber 1g 4%
Protein 5g

---

35 KETO BREAKFAST PIZZA

Prep/Cook Time: 25 minutes

Ingredients:

- 2 cups grated cauliflower
- 2 tablespoons coconut flour
- 1/2 teaspoon salt
- 4 eggs
- 1 tablespoon psyllium husk powder (Use a mold-free brand like this one)
- Toppings: smoked Salmon, avocado, herbs, spinach, olive oil (see post for more suggestions)

Instructions:

- Preheat the oven to 350 degrees. Line a pizza tray or sheet pan with parchment.
- In a mixing bowl, add all ingredients except toppings and mix until combined. Set aside for 5 minutes to allow coconut flour and psyllium husk to absorb liquid and thicken up.
- Carefully pour the breakfast pizza base onto the pan. Use your hands to mold it into a round, even pizza crust.
- Bake for 15 minutes, or until golden brown and fully
- cooked. Remove from the oven and top breakfast pizza with your chosen toppings. Serve warm.

Nutrition Info

Calories: 454
Total Fat: 31g
Saturated Fat: 75g
Net Carbs: 8.8g
Protein: 22g

36 KETO FLAX SEED BREAD

Prep Time 5 minutes
Cook Time 2 minutes
Total Time 7 minutes
Servings 2 Slices

Ingredients

- 1 tablespoon Softened Butter
- 4 tablespoons Organic Ground Flaxseed Meal
- 1 Large Egg
- ½ teaspoon Baking Powder
- ½ teaspoon Salt

Instructions

- Grab your Pyrex glass square dish and add the butter. Melt it in the microwave for a few seconds.
- Crack your egg into the dish and give it a good mix with a
- fork. Mix the ground flax seed, salt and baking powder in a separate bowl and combine.
- Add all the mixed dry ingredients, ground flax, salt, and baking powder directly into the baking dish and combine all ingredients thoroughly.
- It will turn into a thick texture. Flatten out the surface of the mixture to ensure even cooking.
- Cook in the microwave for two minutes.
- Leave to cool for a few minutes before taking out.
- Use a spatula and gently pull the bread away from the side of the dish. After you turn it upside down, it should come out without difficulty.
- Grab your bread knife and cut it in half to make two slices

37 LOW CARB ASPARAGUS EGG BITES

Prep Time: 5 minutes
Cook Time: 15 minutes
Total Time: 20 minutes
Servings: 3

Ingredients

- non-stick cooking spray
- 3 medium asparagus stalks
- 6 eggs
- 1 tbs unsweetened almond milk
- salt and pepper
- 2 tbs grated Parmesan

Instructions

- Preheat the oven to 400F (200C).

- Prepare a six-hole muffin pan by spraying it liberally with some non-stick cooking spray. Chop up the asparagus (to make about half a cup) and divide between the muffin pan cups.

- Beat the eggs and unsweetened almond milk together in a jug. Season with salt and pepper then divide it between the muffin cups.

- Sprinkle some grated Parmesan over the top of each one, then bake in a preheated oven for 12-15 minutes, until golden brown on top and the egg is cooked through. They will puff up while cooking but deflate slightly as they cool.

- Remove the asparagus egg bites from the pan and enjoy warm - or let cool fully and store in the fridge.

Nutrition Info

Calories 143 Calories from Fat 81
Total Fat 9g 14%
Saturated Fat 3g 15%

Sugars 0g
Protein 12g 24%

---

38 LOW SUGAR GLUTEN FREE PUMPKIN BREAD

Prep time: 10 mins
Cook time: 60 mins
Total time: 1 hour 10 mins

Ingredients

- 1 cup coconut flour
- ½ cup Swerve Sweetener, granulated
- 8 eggs (I used large)
- 1 tsp baking soda
- ½ tsp baking powder
- ½ tsp salt
- 1 tsp Sweetleaf Stevia
- 2 tsp cinnamon
- ½ tsp ginger
- 1 tsp ground cloves
- 2 tbsp vanilla extract
- 1 stick butter
- 1, 15-oz can of pureed Pumpkin

Instructions

- Preheat oven to 350 degrees F, and grease a 9x5 bread pan with butter. (Using oil or butter vs spray helps the bread not to stick to the pan.)
- In a large bowl, mix together the dry ingredients of coconut flour, Swerve Sweetener, baking soda, baking powder, salt,

Sweetleaf Stevia, cinnamon, ginger and ground cloves.

- In another bowl, mix together the wet ingredients. When well mixed, add the wet ingredients into the large ingredients and whisk well. (If using a blender, a low-medium blend is fine.)
- Fill the 9x5 bread pan with the pumpkin bread, and bake in the oven until a tooth pick comes out clear. For me, the 50 -1 hr mark was perfect.

39 KETO CHEDDAR BAY BISCUITS

These keto cheddar bay biscuits taste so much like Red Lobster biscuits! Try this copycat recipe for savory, cheesy, and EASY keto dinner rolls.

Prep Time: 5 Mins
Cook Time: 25 Mins
Total Time: 30 mins

Ingredients:

- 2 cups almond flour (what we used)
- 2 teaspoons baking powder
- 1/2 teaspoon Himalayan salt
- 1/2 teaspoon garlic powder
- 1/4 teaspoon ground black pepper
- 4 tablespoons grass-fed unsalted butter, chilled and cut into small pieces
- 4 tablespoons heavy whipping cream
- 2 large eggs, beaten
- 4 ounces white cheddar cheese, shredded

- 2 ounces sharp yellow cheddar cheese, shredded
- 1 tablespoon dried parsley

Instructions

- Preheat oven to 350 degrees. Line a baking sheet with parchment or a silicone baking liner.
- In a large mixing bowl, blend all dry ingredients. Add butter and crumble with a fork (or your hands, if they're cold) until incorporated well into the dry mix.
- Add heavy cream in small amounts, mixing well between each addition. Stir eggs into the mixture. Mix white cheddar into the batter until it forms a doughy consistency, then gently add in yellow cheddar.
- Scoop 8 even portions of dough onto your prepared baking sheet. (You can also roll into balls instead if you want rounder biscuits.)
- Bake for 20 minutes, or until browned on the bottom.
- Serve warm, or cool completely and store in a covered container. Reheat gently in a toaster oven when ready to serve again.

Nutrition Info

Calories 350
Fat (Grams) 32
Sat. Fat (Grams) 12
Carbs (Grams) 6.2

---

40 HEALTHY 3 INGREDIENT MINI PALEO PIZZA BASES CRUSTS

Prep/Cook Time: 50 minutes
Servings: 4
Calories: 125kcal

Ingredients

For the coconut flour option

- 8 large egg whites for thicker bases, use 5 whole eggs and 3 egg whites
- 1/4 cup coconut flour sifted
- 1/2 tsp baking powder
- Spices of choice salt, pepper, Italian spices
- Extra coconut flour to dust very lightly

For the almond flour option

- 8 large egg whites
- 1/2 cup almond flour
- 1/2 tsp baking powder
- Spices of choice salt, pepper, Italian spices

For the pizza sauce

- 1/2 cup Mutti tomato sauce
- 2 cloves garlic crushed
- 1/4 tsp sea salt
- 1 tsp dried basil

Instructions

To make the pizza bases/crusts

- In a large mixing bowl, whisk the eggs/egg whites until opaque. Sift in the coconut flour or almond flour and whisk very well until clumps are removed. Add the baking powder, mixed spices and continue to whisk until completely combined. On low heat, heat
- up a small pan and grease lightly.
- Once frying pan is hot, pour the batter in the pan and ensure it is fully coated. Cover the pan with a lid/tray for 3-4 minutes or until bubbles start to appear on top. Flip, cook for an extra 2 minutes and remove from pan- Keep an eye on this, as it can burn out pretty quickly.
- Continue until all the batter is used up.

- Allow pizza bases to cool. Once cool, use a skewer and poke holes roughly over the top, for even cooking. Dust very lightly with a dash of coconut flour.

To make the sauce

- Combine all the ingredients together and let sit at room temperature for at least 30 minutes- This thickens up.

Nutrition Info

Calories: 125kcal, Carbohydrates: 6g, Protein: 8g, Fat: 1g, Fiber: 3g, Vitamin A: 1%, Vitamin C: 2%, Calcium: 1%, Iron: 2%

41 EASY CLOUD BREAD (NO CREAM CHEESE, LACTOSE-FREE, LOW-CARB, KETO, PALEO)

This oopsie bread is perfect for dairy-free peeps! No cream cheese at all, instead I'm using coconut cream for the same fluffy turnout. These are perfect to make a low carb sandwich, mini pizza, or burger bun!

Prep Time 15 mins
Cook Time 20 mins
Total Time 35 mins
Servings: 10 pieces
Calories: 36 kcal

Ingredients

- 3 eggs
- 3 tbsp coconut cream spoon from refrigerated can of full-fat coconut milk

- 1/2 tsp baking powder
- optional toppings: sea salt black pepper and rosemary or whatever seasonings you like!

Instructions

- Firstly, prep everything. Once you start going, you'll need to move quickly so have everything handy. Pre-heat the oven to 325f degrees and arrange a rack in the middle. Line a baking sheet with parchment paper and set aside. Grab your tools: hand mixer (you can use a stand mixer, but I find it to be better for whipping egg whites so I can stay in control), all ingredients, any additional seasonings, two mixing bowls (the larger one should be used for egg whites), a large spoon to scoop and drop the bread with.
- Using a full-fat can of coconut milk that has been refrigerated overnight or several hours, spoon out the top coconut cream and add to the smaller bowl.
- Separate eggs into the two bowls, adding the yolk to the bowl with the cream and be careful to not let the yolk get into the whites in the larger bowl.
- Using a hand mixer, beat the yolk and cream together first until nice and creamy, make sure there are no clumps of
- coconut left. Wash your whisks well and dry them.
- Add the baking powder into the whites and start beating on medium with the hand mixer for a few minutes, moving around and you'll see it get firmer. Keep going for a few minutes, you want to get it as thick as you can with stiff peaks. The thicker the better. Just don't over-do it. Once you can stop and dip the whisks in leaving peaks behind, you're ready.
- Quickly and carefully add the yolk-coconut mixture into the whites, folding with a spatula, careful not to deflate too much. Keep going until everything is well combined but still fluffy.
- Now you can grab your spoon and start dropping your batter down on the baking sheet. Keep going as quickly and carefully as you can, or it will start to melt. They should look pillow-y.
- Steadily add your baking sheet to the middle rack in the oven and bake for approx. 20-25 minutes. You should be able to

scoop them up with your spatula and see a fluffy top and a flat bottom. Store in the fridge for about a week or freeze.

42 SIMPLE AND FLUFFY GLUTEN-FREE LOW-CARB BREAD

Prep/Cook Time: 50 minutes

Ingredients

- 1/2 cup = 120 ml = 45 g unflavored whey protein
- powder 2 teaspoons aluminium-free baking powder
- 1/2 cup = 120 ml = 125 g almond butter (natural,
- unsweetened) 4 extra large organic eggs

Intructions

- Preheat the oven to 300 °F (150 °C).
- Mix well the whey protein and baking powder in a small
- bowl. Beat the almond butter with an electric mixer in a large bowl until creamy.
- Add one egg at a time beating well after each addition until the batter is smooth, fluffy and bubbly.
- Combine the whey protein mixture with the almond butter mixture and beat well until creamy.
- Pour the batter in a 9 X 5 inch (23 X 13 cm) silicone loaf pan.
- Bake for 30–40 minutes.
- Let cool, remove from the pan and cut into slices.

43 LOW CARB PALEO TORTILLAS RECIPE - 3 INGREDIENT COCONUT FLOUR WRAPS

If you're looking for easy coconut flour recipes, try paleo low carb tortillas with coconut flour. Just 3 ingredients in these keto paleo coconut wraps!

Prep Time 5 minutes
Cook Time 10 minutes
Total Time 15 minutes
Servings 8" tortillas

Ingredients

- 1/2 cup Coconut flour
- 6 large Eggs (up to 7-8, see notes)
- 1 1/4 cup Unsweetened almond milk (up to 1 1/2 cup, see notes; can also use any milk of choice - use coconut milk beverage for nut-free)
- 3/4 tsp Sea salt (optional)
- 1 tbsp Gelatin powder (optional - for more pliable, sturdy tortillas)
- 1/2 tsp Cumin (optional)
- 1/2 tsp Paprika (optional)

Instructions

- In a large bowl, whisk all ingredients together until smooth. Let the batter sit for a minute or two to account for the natural thickening caused by coconut flour. The batter should be very runny right before cooking - it should pour easily (add more almond milk and eggs in *equal* proportions if needed to achieve this). If you are using the optional gelatin, add an extra 1/4 cup almond milk.

- Heat a small skillet (about 8 in (20 cm) diameter) over medium to medium-high heat and grease lightly (use oil of choice or an oil mister). Pour 1/4 cup (60 mL) of batter onto the skillet and immediately, rapidly tilt in different directions to evenly distribute, like making crepes. Cook, covered with a lid, until the edges are golden and you see bubbles forming in the middle. The edges will curl inward when you lift the lid (about 1-2 minutes). Flip over, cover again, and cook until browned on the other side (1-2 more minutes). Repeat until the batter is used up.

Nutrition Info

Calories 55
Fat 3g
Protein 5g
Total Carbs 4g
Net Carbs 1g
Fiber 3g
Sugar 1g

44 PEANUT BUTTER BERRY BREAKFAST LOAF

Serving: 12 Slices

Ingredients

- 1/2 cup peanut butter
- 1/4 cup grass fed butter, melted

- 5 pastured eggs
- 1/2 cup coconut milk or almond milk
- 1 tsp vanilla extract
- 1/2 cup almond flour
- 3 tbsp Swerve sweetener (more for a sweeter bread) (I get it here)
- 2 tsp baking powder
- 1/2 tsp sea salt
- 1/2 cup frozen mixed berries

Instructions

- Preheat oven to 350°. Use a silicone loaf pan (Get one here) or line a loaf pan with parchment paper.
- In a large mixing bowl, combine peanut butter, melted butter and eggs. Mix until well combined.
- Add the coconut milk and vanilla extract and mix to combine.
- In a separate mixing bowl, combine the almond flour, sweetener, baking powder and sea salt. mix together until well combined and all chunks of baking powder are broken up.
- Slowly pour the wet mixture into the dry ingredients, mixing as you pour.
- Mix until all ingredients are well incorporated.
- Using a rubber spatula, gently fold the mixed berries into the mixture.
- Pour the batter evenly into the loaf pan.
- Bake for 45 minutes to an hour, checking on it at the 45 minute mark.
- Remove from oven and allow to cool before slicing.
- Pop a couple slices in the toaster and then slather them with delicious grass fed butter!

Nutrition Info

Calories: 153, Fat: 13g, Protein: 5.8g, Total Carbs: 4.83g, Fiber: 1.5g, Net Carbs: 3.33g

45 LEMON POPPY SEED LOAF CAKE

Prep Time 10 mins
Cook Time 1 hr
Total Time 1 hr 10 mins
Servings: 12

Ingredients

- 2/3 cup cottage cheese
- 4 tbsp butter softened
- 1/2 cup Trim Healthy Mama Gentle Sweet or my
- sweetener 4 eggs
- 3 tbsp lemon juice
- 1 1/2 cup almond flour
- 1/2 cup coconut flour
- 2 tsp baking powder
- 1 tsp lemon zest
- 2 tbsp poppy seeds

Instructions

- Preheat oven to 350. Grease a standard loaf pan well with cooking spray.

- Combine the cottage cheese, butter, and sweetener in the food processor. Pulse until smooth. Add the eggs, lemon juice, flours, baking powder, and zest. Pulse until well combined. Add the poppy seeds and pulse until they are evenly distributed in the batter. Transfer the batter to the prepared loaf pan.

- Bake for 55-65 min or until the center feels firm when lightly pressed and the edges are deep golden brown.

- Cool completely to make it easier to remove from the pan. Alternatively, you can line the loaf pan with parchment paper.

Nutrition Info

Calories 176 Calories from Fat 117

Total Fat 13g 20%
Saturated Fat 4g 20%
Cholesterol 66mg 22%
Sodium 108mg 5%
Potassium 130mg 4%
Total Carbohydrates 7g 2%
Dietary Fiber 3g 12%
Sugars 1g
Protein 7g 14%

---

46 PALEO CHOCOLATE ZUCCHINI BREAD

Prep Time10 mins
Cook Time50 mins
Cool down4 hrs
Total Time1 hr
Servings: 12 slices
Calories: 185kcal

Ingredients

Dry ingredients

- 1 1/2 cup almond flour (170g)
- 1/4 cup unsweetened cocoa powder (25g)
- 1 1/2 teaspoon baking soda
- 2 teaspoons ground cinnamon
- 1/4 teaspoon sea salt
- 1/2 cup sugar free crystal sweetener (Monk fruit or erythritol) (100g) or coconut sugar if refined sugar free

Wet ingredients

- 1 cup zucchini, finely grated measure packed, discard juice/liquid if there is some - about 2 small zucchini
- 1 large egg
- 1/4 cup + 2 tablespoon canned coconut cream
- 100ml 1/4 cup extra virgin coconut oil , melted, 60ml

- 1 teaspoon vanilla extract
- 1 teaspoon apple cider vinegar

Filling - optional

- 1/2 cup sugar free chocolate chips
- 1/2 cup chopped walnuts or nuts you like

Instructions

- Preheat oven to 180C (375F). Line a baking loaf pan (9 inches x 5 inches) with parchment paper. Set aside.
- Remove both extremity of the zucchinis, keep skin on.
- Finely grate the zucchini using a vegetable grater. Measure the amount needed in a measurement cup. Make sure you press/pack them firmly for a precise measure and to squeeze out any liquid from the grated zucchini, I usually don't have any!. If you do, discard the liquid or keep for another recipe.
- In a large mixing bowl, stir all the dry ingredients together: almond flour, unsweetened cocoa powder, sugar free crystal sweetener, cinnamon, sea salt and baking soda. Set aside.
- Add all the wet ingredients into the dry ingredients : grated zucchini, coconut oil, coconut cream, vanilla, egg, apple cider vinegar.
- Stir to combine all the ingredients together.
- Stir in the chopped nuts and sugar free chocolate chips.
- Transfer the chocolate bread batter into the prepared loaf
- pan. Bake 50 - 55 minutes, you may want to cover the bread loaf with a piece of foil after 40 minute to avoid the top to darken too much, up to you.
- The bread will stay slightly moist in the middle and firm up after fully cool down.

Cool down

- Cool down 10 minutes in the loaf pan, then cool down on a cooling rack until it reach room temperature. It can take 4 hours as it is a thick bread. Don' slice the bread before it reach room temperature. If too hot in the center, it will be too oft and fall apart when you slice. For a faster result, cool down 40 minutes at room temperature then pop in the fridge for 1 hour. The fridge will create an extra fudgy texture and the bread will be even easier to slice as it firms up.

- Store in the fridge up to 4 days in a cake bow or airtight container.

Nutrition Info

Calories: 185kcal, Carbohydrates: 6.1g, Protein: 4.9g, Fat: 17.1g, Fiber: 2.7g, Sugar: 1.2g

47 ROSEMARY AND GARLIC COCONUT FLOUR BREAD

Prep Time: 10 minutes
Cook Time: 45 minutes
Total Time: 55 minutes
Servings: 10 Slices

Ingredients

- 1/2 cup Coconut flour
- 1 stick butter (8 tbsp)
- 6 large eggs
- 1 tsp Baking powder
- 2 tsp Dried Rosemary
- 1/2-1 tsp garlic powder

- 1/2 tsp Onion powder
- 1/4 tsp Pink Himalayan Salt

Instructions

-
- Combine dry ingredients (coconut flour, baking powder, onion, garlic, rosemary and salt) in a bowl and set aside.
- Add 6 eggs to a separate bowl and beat with a hand mixer until you get see bubbles at the top.
- Melt the stick of butter in the microwave and slowly add it to the eggs as you beat with the hand mixer.
- Once wet and dry ingredients are fully combined in separate bowls, slowly add the dry ingredients to the wet ingredients as you mix with the hand mixture.
- Grease an 8x4 loaf pan and pour the mixture into it
- evenly. Bake at 350 for 40-50 minutes (time will vary depending on your oven).
- Let it rest for 10 minutes before removing from the pan. Slice up and enjoy with butter or toasted!

Nutrition Info

Calories: 147kcal, Carbohydrates: 3.5g, Protein: 4.6g, Fat: 12.5g, Fiber: 2g

48 COCONUT FLOUR PSYLLIUM HUSK BREAD - PALEO

Want an easy low carb keto Paleo bread? Try this gluten free coconut flour psyllium bread recipe. It's a tasty bread to serve with breakfast or dinner.

Prep Time 5 minutes
Cook Time 55 minutes

Total Time 1 hour
Servings 15 slices
Calories 127kcal

Ingredients

- 6 tablespoons whole psyllium husks 27g, may want to finely grind
- 3/4 cup warm water
- 1 cup coconut flour 125g
- 1 1/2 teaspoons baking soda
- 3/4 teaspoon sea salt
- 1 pint egg whites 2 cups (or use 8 whole eggs)
- 2 large eggs see note
- 1/2 cup olive oil
- 1/4 cup coconut oil melted

Instructions

- Preheat oven to 350°F.
- If not using silicone pan, grease or line pan with parchment paper. I used an 8x4-in pan.
- Dump all ingredients into a food processor and pulse until well combined. If you don't have a food processor, you can use a mixing bowl with electric mixer.
- Spread batter into 8x4 loaf pan. Smooth top.
- Bake for 45-55 minutes or until edges are brown and toothpick inserted comes out clean.
- Let bread sit in pan for 15 minutes. Remove bread from pan and allow to cool completely on rack.

Nutrition Info

Calories 127
Calories from Fat 120
Total Fat 13.3g 20%
Protein 3g 6%

49 KETO FATHEAD BAGELS

Prep Time 20 mins
Cook Time 20 mins
Total Time 40 mins
Servings: 8 servings

Ingredients

- 1/2 cup coconut flour (56g)
- 2 tsp baking powder
- 3/4 tsp xanthan gum
- 12 oz pre-shredded part skim mozzarella
- 2 large eggs

Optional Topping for Everything Bagels

- 1 tsp sesame seeds
- 1 tsp poppyseed
- 1 tsp dried minced onion
- 1/2 tsp coarse salt
- 1 tbsp butter melted

Instructions

- Preheat the oven to 350F and line a large baking sheet with a silicone liner. In a medium bowl, whisk together the coconut flour, baking powder, and xanthan gum. Set aside.

- In a large microwave safe bowl, melt the cheese on high in 30 second increments until well melted and almost liquid. Stir in the flour mixture and the eggs and knead in the bowl using a rubber spatula.

- Turn out onto the prepared baking sheet and continue to knead together until cohesive. Cut the dough in half and cut each half into 4 equal portions so that you have 8 equal pieces of dough.

- Roll each portion out into a log about 8 inches long. Pinch the ends of the log together.

- In a shallow dish, stir together the sesame seeds, poppyseed, dried onion, and salt. Brush the top of each bagel with melted butter and dip firmly into the everything seasoning. Set back on the silicone mat.

- Bake 15 to 20 minutes, until the bagels have risen and are golden brown.

Nutrition Info

Calories 190 Calories from Fat 111
Total Fat 12.3g 19%
Total Carbohydrates 5.5g 2%
Dietary Fiber 2.6g 10%
Protein 12.1g 24%

50 (15 MINUTE!) GLUTEN FREE & KETO PIZZA CRUST

Prep Time: 10 minutes
Cook Time: 5 minutes
Total Time: 15 minutes
Servings: slices
Calories: 118 kcal

Ingredients

For the keto pizza dough:

- 96 g almond flour
- 24 g coconut flour
- 2 teaspoons xanthan gum
- 2 teaspoons baking powder
- 1/4 teaspoon kosher salt depending on whether sweet or savory
- 2 teaspoons apple cider vinegar
- 1 egg lightly beaten
- 5 teaspoons water as needed

Topping suggestions:

- our keto marinara sauce
- mozzarella cheese
- pepperoni or salami
- fresh basil

Instructions

For the keto dough:

- Add almond flour, coconut flour, xanthan gum, baking powder and salt to food processor. Pulse until thoroughly combined.

- Pour in apple cider vinegar with the food processor running. Once it has distributed evenly, pour in the egg. Followed by the water, adding just enough for it to come together into a ball. The dough will be sticky to touch from the xanthan gum, but still sturdy.

- Wrap dough in plastic wrap and knead it through the plastic for a minute or two. Think of it a bit like a stress ball. The dough should be smooth and not significantly cracked (a couple here and there are fine). In which case get it back to the food processor and add in more water 1 teaspoon at a time. Allow dough to rest for 10 minutes at room temperature (and up to 5 days in the fridge).

- If cooking on the stove top: heat up a skillet or pan over medium/high heat while your dough rests (you want the pan to be very hot!). If using the oven: heat up a pizza stone, skillet or baking tray in the oven at 350°F/180°C. The premise is that you need to blind cook/bake the crust first on both sides without toppings on a very hot surface.

- Roll out dough between two sheets of parchment paper with a rolling pin. You can play with thickness here, but we like to roll it out nice and thin (roughly 12 inches in diameter) and fold over the edges (pressing down with wet fingertips).

- Cook the pizza crust in your pre-heated skillet or pan, top-side down first, until blistered (about 2 minutes, depending on your skillet and heat). Lower heat to medium/low, flip over your pizza crust, add toppings of choice and cover with a lid. Alternatively you can always transfer it to your oven on grill to finish off the pizza.

- Serve right away. Alternatively, note that the dough can be kept in the fridge for about 5 days. So you can make individual mini pizzettes throughout the week.

Nutrition Info

Calories 118 Calories from Fat 81
Total Fat 9g 14%
Saturated Fat 1.3g 7%
Cholesterol 27mg 9%
Dietary Fiber 3g 12%
Sugars 0.8g
Protein 5g 10%

51 ROSEMARY AND GARLIC COCONUT FLOUR BREAD

Prep Time: 10 minutes
Cook Time: 45 minutes
Total Time: 55 minutes
Servings: 10 Slices

Ingredients

- 1/2 cup Coconut flour
- 1 stick butter (8 tbsp)
- 6 large eggs
- 1 tsp Baking powder
- 2 tsp Dried Rosemary
- 1/2-1 tsp garlic powder
- 1/2 tsp Onion powder
- 1/4 tsp Pink Himalayan Salt

Instructions

- Combine dry ingredients (coconut flour, baking powder, onion, garlic, rosemary and salt) in a bowl and set aside.
- Add 6 eggs to a separate bowl and beat with a hand mixer until you get see bubbles at the top.
- Melt the stick of butter in the microwave and slowly add it to the eggs as you beat with the hand mixer.
- Once wet and dry ingredients are fully combined in separate bowls, slowly add the dry ingredients to the wet ingredients as you mix with the hand mixture.
- Grease an 8x4 loaf pan and pour the mixture into it evenly.
- Bake at 350 for 40-50 minutes (time will vary depending on your oven).
- Let it rest for 10 minutes before removing from the pan. Slice up and enjoy with butter or toasted!

Nutrition Info

Calories: 147kcal, Carbohydrates: 3.5g, Protein: 4.6g, Fat: 12.5g, Fiber: 2g

52 KETO + LOW CARB CORNBREAD MUFFINS

Prep Time: 15 minutes
Cook Time: 25 minutes
Total Time: 40 minutes
Servings: 12

Ingredients

- 3 eggs, slightly beaten
- 1/2 cup heavy whipping cream
- 1/2 cup unsweetened coconut milk (from a carton, not a jar)
- 5 tbsp salted butter, melted
- 3 oz cream cheese, softened
- 1 cup (128g) coconut flour
- 1/4 cup (30g) almond meal
- 3 tbsp (27g) Swerve Confectioners
- 1 1/2 tsp baking powder
- 1/8 tsp salt

Instructions

- Pre-heat oven to 350 F.
- If you're using a silicone muffin pan like I did, you don't need to grease the pan. However, if you're not using silicone, I recommend lightly greasing it or using liners for easy
- removal. In a large bowl, combine eggs, heavy whipping cream, coconut milk, melted butter (cooled slightly), and cream cheese. Using a hand mixer, mix everything until the cream cheese is well-incorporated. (It's okay if you have a few small flecks remaining.) Set aside.
- In a medium-sized bowl, combine coconut flour, almond meal, Swerve Confectioners, baking powder, and salt. Mix thoroughly.
- Add dry ingredients to wet and mix thoroughly using your hand mixer.
- Evenly distribute the batter across the holes, pressing the batter down a bit with the back of a spoon. (The batter is thick and easily forms pockets.) They will be about 80% full.

- Place in the oven and bake for 20-25 minutes until the edges start to brown and an inserted toothpick comes out mostly clean. Do not overbake. The center should still be slightly soft (but not uncooked) when you pull the pan out of the oven.
- of the oven. Cool and enjoy!

Nutrition Info

Calories 169 Calories from Fat 126
Total Fat 14g 22%
Sugars 0g
Protein 4g 8%

---

53 LOW CARB FOCACCIA BREAD

Prep Time15 mins
Cook Time30 mins
Total Time45 mins
Servings: Loaf

Ingredients

- 50 g coconut flour
- 5 tbsp psyllium husk
- 2 tsp baking powder
- 1 tsp salt
- 4 eggs - medium
- 250 ml boiling water

Instructions

- Place the coconut flour, psyllium husks, baking powder and salt into a large mixing bowl and stir until combined.
- Add the eggs and mix. The mixture will be a very firm 'play-dough' like consistency so don't work it too hard at
- this point. Add the cup of boiling water and mix until thoroughly combined.
- Form into a focaccia shape and place on a baking tray lined with baking paper. Using a sharp knife, make diagonal cuts

through the dough, sprinkle with plenty of salt, rosemary and place olives on top of the dough.

- Bake at 180C for 25-30 minutes. It is cooked when the centre is no longer 'spongy'.
- Serve hot with butter, cold with cheese, avocado slices, tomatoes, labna, etc.

Nutrition Info

Calories 528 Calories from Fat 234
Total Fat 26g 40%
Total Carbohydrates 58g 19%
Dietary Fiber 42g 168%
Sugars 5.9g
Protein 31g 62%

54 KETO CRANBERRY ORANGE BREAD

Prep Time: 10 minutes
Cook Time: 1 hour
Additional Time: 10 minutes
Total Time: 1 hour 20 minutes
Serving: 12

Ingredients

Keto Cranberry Orange Bread Batter

- 2 1/2 cups of finely milled almond flour
- 1 cup of sugar substitute
- 2 teaspoons of baking powder
- 1/2 teaspoon of sea salt

- 8 whole eggs
- 8 ounces of room temperature full-fat cream cheese
- 2 teaspoons of orange extract
- 1/2 cup of room temperature unsalted
- butter 2 cups of fresh or frozen whole
- cranberries 1 tablespoon of orange zest

Keto Orange Glaze

- 3/4 cup of confectioners sugar substitute
- 3 tablespoons of freshly squeezed lemon juice
- 2 tablespoons of heavy whipping cream
- 1 teaspoon of orange extract
- 2 teaspoons of orange zest

Instructions

Keto Cranberry Orange Bread

- Preheat oven to 350 degrees.
- Grease and line with parchment paper a 10 inch loaf pan or two 6 inch loaf pans. (note if using two smaller pans check for doneness at 35 minute mark)
- In a medium-sized bowl measure then sift the almond flour. To the sifted flour add the baking powder, sea salt and stir. Set this aside.
- In a large bowl using an electric hand-held mixer or stand-up mixer blend the butter, cream cheese, and sugar-substitute until mixture is light fluffy.
- Next add the eggs one at a time, making sure to scrape the bowl several times.
- To the wet batter add the dry ingredients and combine until well-incorporated.
- Fold in the cranberries in the bread batter.
- Spread the batter into the greased loaf pan.
- Bake for 60-70 minutes or until an inserted toothpick comes out clean.
- Allow the loaf to cool in the pan for about 30 minutes before taking it out of the pan. Then let the pan cool on a baking rack

for another 30 minutes before adding the icing or freezing.

Keto Orange Icing

- In a small mixing bowl whisk the confectioners sugar substitute, lemon juice, orange zest, orange extract and heavy cream. Stir until fully combined.
- Spread/drizzle the icing over the cooled keto cranberry bread.

Nutrition Info

Calories: 337 Total Fat: 30.6g Saturated Fat: 11.4g Cholesterol: 154mg Sodium: 157mg Carbohydrates: 6.9g Fiber: 3.2g Sugar: 1.9g Protein: 10.3g

55 LOW CARB CARROT CAKE MUFFINS

This low carb carrot cake muffins are great for snacking! Sugar free, gluten free, and keto recipe.

Prep Time: 10 minutes
Cook Time: 25 minutes
Cooling Time: 5 minutes
Total Time: 35 minutes
Servings: 6

Ingredients

- 1 carrot peeled and grated
- 1 cup almond flour
- 3 eggs
- ¼ cup melted butter
- 2 tbs low carb sweetener eg Swerve
- ½ tsp baking powder
- ½ tsp vanilla extract

Instructions

- Preheat the oven to 350F (175C).

- In a stand mixer bowl, add almond flour, eggs, melted butter, sweetener, baking powder and vanilla extract. Blend until fully combined.
- Stir in the grated carrot until mixed through the batter.
- Divide the mixture between a six-hole muffin pan that has been lined with paper or silicone liners.
- Bake in a preheated oven for 20-25 minutes or until cooked through. Let cool for 5 minutes before serving.

Nutrition Info

Calories 210 Calories from Fat 171
Total Fat 19g 29%
Saturated Fat 6g 30%
Dietary Fiber 2g 8%
Sugars 1g

---

56 CHEDDAR GARLIC FATHEAD ROLLS

Prep Time 10 mins
Cook Time 25 mins
Total Time 35 mins
Servings: 8 servings

Ingredients

Rolls:

- 8 ounces cheddar cheese grated (I used Cabot Vermont Cheddar)
- 2 tbsp butter
- 1/2 cup coconut flour
- 1/4 cup unflavored whey protein powder or egg white protein

powder
- 4 tsp baking powder
- 1 tsp garlic powder
- 1/4 tsp salt
- 2 large eggs
- 1 large egg white

Garlic Butter

- 2 tbsp butter melted
- 2 cloves garlic minced
- 1 tbsp chopped parsley
- 1/2 tsp coarse salt

Instructions

- Preheat the oven to 350F and line an 8-inch round baking pan with parchment paper.

- In a large microwave safe bowl, combine the grated cheese and the butter. Melt on high in 30 second increments until the cheese and butter can be stirred together and is almost liquid.

- Add the coconut flour, protein powder, baking powder, garlic powder, and salt. Stir in the eggs and egg white and use a rubber spatula to "knead" together in the bowl until uniform.

- Divide the dough into 8 equal portions. The dough will be quite sticky so lightly oil your hands and roll into 8 ball. Place in the prepared baking pan.

- Whisk together the ingredients for the garlic butter and brush about half of it over the rolls in the pan.

- Bake 20 to 25 minutes, until puffed, golden brown, and firm to the touch. Remove and let cool about15 minutes before removing from the pan and breaking apart. Brush with the remaining garlic butter. Serve warm.

Nutrition Info

Calories 230 Calories from Fat 143
Total Fat 15.9g 24%
Total Carbohydrates 5.9g 2%
Dietary Fiber 2.6g 10%
Protein 12.2g 24%

---

57 3 MINUTE LOW CARB BISCUITS

Prep Time: 2 minutes
Cook Time: 3 minutes
Total Time: 5 minutes
Servings: 1 Servings
Calories: 392kcal

Ingredients

- 1 tbsp Butter
- 2 tbsp Coconut flour
- 1 large Egg
- 1 tbsp Heavy Whipping Cream
- 2 tbsp Water
- 1/4 cup Cheddar Cheese
- 1/8 tsp garlic powder
- 1/8 tsp Onion powder
- 1/8 tsp Dried Parsley

- 1/8 tsp Pink Himalayan Salt
- 1/8 tsp black pepper
- 1/4 tsp Baking powder

Instructions

- Melt butter in a coffee mug by microwaving for 20
- seconds. Add coconut flour, baking powder, and seasonings. Mix to incorporate with a fork.
- Add egg, water, cheese and heavy whipping cream. Mix until combined.
- Microwave for 3 minutes. Immediately remove from mug and allow to cool for 2 minutes.
- Slice and enjoy.

Nutrition Info

Calories: 392kcal, Carbohydrates: 9g, Protein: 15g, Fat: 32g, Fiber: 5g

---

58 HOMEMADE NUT AND SEED PALEO BREAD

Prep Time: 10 min
Cook Time: 40 min
Total Time: 50 minutes
Serving: 12 -15 slices

Ingredients

- 1 1/4 cup almond flour
- 5 eggs (6 if you want extra fluffy)

- 1/3 cup coconut oil or avocado oil
- 1 tsp white vinegar or apple cider
- vinegar 1/2 tsp sea salt
- dash of black pepper
- Optional 1 tsp spice mix of choice (garlic, rosemary, Italian, etc.).
- 1 – 2 tsp poppyseed (plus extra for topping)
- 3 to 4 tbsp tapioca flour (if you are using more egg, add 4
- tbsp). 1/2 tsp baking soda
- 1/4 cup chia meal (just grind chia seed in a coffee grinder or blender) or use ground flaxseed
- Pumpkin seed for topping and Extra poppyseed

Instructions

- Preheat oven to 350. Grease a 9×5 bread pan or line with parchment paper. Set aside. For higher rising bread, use an 8×4 pan.
- In a small bowl, whisk your eggs, oil, and vinegar.
- In another bowl, combine your flours, poppyseed, and seasonings.
- Add your wet ingredients to dry ingredients and mix thoroughly.
- Pour batter into greased pan and top with additional pumpkin seeds and and additional poppyseed.
- Bake covered for 20 minutes. Then uncover and continue to bake for additional 15-20 more or golden and knife in the centre comes out clean.
- Should be around 35-45 minutes all together depending on your oven. If you used 8×4 or are baking at higher elevation, you might need to bake longer.
- Remove from oven and let cool.
- Wrap the paleo bread in foil or plastic wrap, slice and store in container. Keeps well in fridge for up to 7 days or freezer for up to 3 months.

59 HOT HAM AND CHEESE ROLL-UPS WITH DIJON BUTTER GLAZE

Prep/Cook Time: 40 minutes

Servings: 4

Ingredients

For the Hot Ham and Cheese Roll-Ups

- 1/4 cup almond flour (get it here)
- 3 tablespoons coconut flour (get it here)
- 1 teaspoon onion powder
- 1 teaspoon garlic powder
- 1 1/2 cup low-moisture, part skim mozzarella cheese, shredded
- 4 tablespoons salted butter
- 2 tablespoons cream cheese
- 1 large pastured egg
- 10 ounces sliced ham
- 1 1/2 cups sharp white cheddar cheese, shredded

For the Dijon Butter Glaze

- 2 tablespoons salted butter
- 1 tablespoon Dijon mustard
- 1 teaspoon Worcestershire sauce
- 1 teaspoon garlic powder
- 1/2 teaspoon dried Italian seasoning

Instructions

- Preheat oven to 375°F.
- In a small mixing bowl, combine almond flour, coconut flour, onion powder and garlic powder.
- In a separate mixing bowl, combine mozzarella cheese, butter, and cream cheese. Microwave for 1 minute and 30 seconds to soften. Mix together until everything is well combined. If if

gets stringy or is not quite melted enough, put it back in for another 30 seconds.

- To the cheese mixture, add the dry ingredients and the egg. Mix until all ingredients are well incorporated. If you are having a hard time mixing it, put it back in the microwave for another 20-30 seconds.
- Once the ingredients are combined, spread the dough out on parchment paper or a silpat in a thin and even layer – about 9 1/2 by 13 1/2. If it starts to get sticky, wet your hands a little bit to prevent it from sticking to you.
- Once you have the dough in a nice, even rectangle, sprinkle the cheddar over top, covering all of the dough.
- Next, layer on the ham.
- Roll the dough up tightly lengthwise. This will produce smaller rolls, but you will get almost twice as many. Turn so that the seam is facing down
- Cut the ends off each side of the roll-up to even it out. Then cut it into 1 1/2 slices.
- Place your individual roll-ups in a baking dish.
- Bake for 20-25 minutes or until they are fluffy and golden brown.
- While they are baking, melt the butter and mix it with the Dijon, Worcestershire, garlic powder and Italian seasoning. Fork whisk until all ingredients are well incorporated.
- Take your rolls out of the oven, brush the glaze over top of them. Return them to the oven and bake for an additional 5 minutes.

Nutrition Info

Calories – 482 , Fat – 41g , Protein – 25g. , Carbs – 6.8g , Fiber – 2.8g, Net Carbs – 4g

---

60 NEARLY NO CARB KETO BREAD

Prep Time 10 minutes

Cook Time 21 minutes
Total Time 31 minutes
Servings 12 people

Ingredients

- 8 ounces cream cheese
- 2 cups mozzarella cheese grated (about 210 grams)
- 3 large eggs
- 1/4 cup parmesan cheese grated (about 27 grams)
- 1 cup crushed pork rinds about 46 grams
- 1 tablespoon baking powder

Optional:

- herbs and spices to taste

Instructions

- Preheat oven to 375°F. Line baking sheet (I used a 12 x 17 jelly roll pan) with parchment paper.
- Place cream cheese and mozzarella cheese in large microwaveable bowl.
- Microwave cheese on high power for one minute, stir, then microwave for another minute and stir again. The cheese should be fully melted.
- Add egg, parmesan, pork rinds, and baking powder. Stir until all ingredients have been incorporated.
- Spread mixture onto parchment paper lined pan. Bake at 375°F for 15-20 or until lightly brown on top.
- Allow pan to cool on rack for 15 minutes, then remove bread from pan and cool directly on rack.
- Slice into 12 equal sized pieces. Can be eaten plain or used to make sandwiches.

Nutrition Info

Calories 166 Calories from Fat 117
Total Fat 13g 20%
Sugars 0g

Protein 9g 18%

CONCLUSION

The bottom line is that ketogenic diets are very effective for burning body fat, as long as they are done correctly. Ketogenic dieting defies scientific rationale, and there is still a great deal unknown about the long-term effects of low-carbohydrate dieting. Research it, and you might find that it's right for you when the next pre-contest diet begins!

CPSIA information can be obtained
at www.ICGtesting.com
Printed in the USA
LVHW100805120521
687184LV00006B/631